Adult Religious Education as Transformative Learning

The Use of Religious Coping Strategies as a Response to Stress

DR. DETRA BISHOP

WESTBOW
PRESS®
A DIVISION OF THOMAS NELSON
& ZONDERVAN

WestBow Press books may be ordered through booksellers or by contacting:

WestBow Press
A Division of Thomas Nelson & Zondervan
1663 Liberty Drive
Bloomington, IN 47403
www.westbowpress.com
1 (866) 928-1240

ISBN: 978-1-9736-7120-6 (sc)
ISBN: 978-1-9736-7121-3 (e)

Print information available on the last page.

WestBow Press rev. date: 8/19/2019

ABSTRACT
ADULT RELIGIOUS EDUCATION AS TRANSFORMATIVE LEARNING:
THE USE OF RELIGIOUS COPING STRATEGIES AS A RESPONSE TO STRESS

by Detra Bishop

Dissertation, December 2006

The purpose of this study was to explore the relationship between participation in adult religious education and coping resources used by African-American women and to determine if there was a relationship between stressful life events, certain demographic variables, and the use of coping resources. A total of 126 women from Protestant churches in southeast Mississippi were surveyed using the Religious Participation Assessment (RPA), the Social Readjustment Rating Scale (SRRS), the Coping Resources Inventory (CRI), and the Ways of Religious Coping Scale (WORCS). Five women participated in a follow-up interview.

Pearson correlation analyses indicated positive linear relationships between RPA and CRI and RPA and WORCS; coping scores increased in proportion to level of participation in religious activities. Multiple regression analyses exploring the relationship between the experience of stressful life events, the use of coping resources, and demographic variables revealed only one statistically significant finding: stressful events decreased as age increased. Results from qualitative data collected from interviews revealed that church involvement, reading the Bible, and prayer all played a major role in transforming and sustaining these women's lives following a disorienting dilemma. In conclusion, the results from this study suggest that participation in adult religious education is a significant coping strategy for African-American women.

DEDICATION

Bless the LORD, O my soul:
and all that is within me,
bless his holy name.
Bless the LORD, O my soul,
and forget not all his benefits:
Who forgiveth all thine iniquities;
who healeth all thy diseases;
Who redeemeth thy life from destruction;
who crowneth thee with lovingkindness
and tender mercies;
Who satisfieth thy mouth with good things;
so that thy youth is renewed like the eagle's. (Psalm 103:1-5)

I dedicate this published work to my mother (the late Annie Laura), my daughter (Rasheeda), and all other family members who supported me in aspiration to become an author. And God knows I would have been lost without the support of my close friends, prayer partners, and church families, and my beloved mentor (the late Reverend Dr. Ralph Woullard, Jr.). Last, but definitely not least, I acknowledge the prophetic push of my late Uncle George Bishop. Uncle George always called me "the philosopher." Thank you, Uncle George. We made it. God bless you all!

ACKNOWLEDGEMENTS

I offer my deepest gratitude to the members of my committee for their patience and support throughout the dissertation process. Also, I am most honored to have had Dr. Paulette Isaac-Savage as my mentor, who lovingly critiqued and encouraged me all the way. My sincere appreciation is extended to Dr. Lin Harper, my confidant and longtime friend, for pushing me to get focused and stay focused. I am especially grateful to those copyright holders who allowed me to adapt and reprint their survey instruments that were used in the original research: (1) SRRS, Rich Scott and Elsevier, Inc., (2) CRI, M. Susan Marting and Allen Hammer, and (3) WORCS, Dr. Edwin Boudreaux.

CONTENTS

LIST OF TABLES

CHAPTER I
INTRODUCTION

Background

This study is grounded in the perspective transformation theory. The impact of adult religious education and life events on coping strategies are viewed from the standpoint of transformative learning. According to Mezirow and Associates (2000), a "micro-orientation to transformative learning helps bring to light related complexities that have been overlooked in the general trend of studies that focus on perspective transformation in relation to different life events" (p. 318). In consideration of the "micro-orientation" approach, this current study examined of how African-American women's choices of coping strategies were influenced by stressful life events, religious culture, and various demographics factors—assuming a transformative adult religious education learning environment that is founded on faith in God.

Researchers and historians have well documented the fact that people, especially disenfranchised people, rely on faith in God to see them through tough times (Graham, Furr, Flowers, & Burke, 2001; Pargament, 1997; Walsh, 1999). According to Walsh, "There has been a resurging interest in religion and spirituality at the close of the 20th century as people have sought greater meaning, harmony, and connection in their lives" (p. 4). In fact, throughout American history religion has been the center of African-American culture (DuBois, 1989; Ellison & Gay, 1990; Pargament, 1997). At the time of Walsh's study, he found that "more than 90% of Americans identified with a specific religion" (p. 12). Even today, our country remains predominantly Christian (85%). However, there has been a shift in various denominations.

Reportedly, African-Americans are the most religious people (Chatters, Levin, & Taylor, 1992). Therefore, it is not surprising that the African-American church has played a significant role in their lives. According to Isaac (2005), "Historically, the African American church has provided educational training and personal development for African American adults" (p. 280). Interestingly, Pargament (1997) noted that religious institutions like the African-American church are well positioned to aid at-risk and disenfranchised groups in our society. The African-American church in many instances serves a full range of physical, social, and spiritual needs, which are preventable in nature.

Tisdale (2000) embraced the holistic aspect of religion/spirituality. She conducted a qualitative study that explored how "spirituality influences the motivations and practices of a multicultural group of 16 women adult educators" (p. 308). In this study, she also indicates how religion/spirituality has a holistic effect on the lives of the women in her study.

Although all the women in Tisdale's (2000) study reported having had "personal experiences of marginalization" (p. 316), only nine were actually women of color. All of the women discussed crucial times in their lives when they "had a strong sense of a divine presence that facilitated healing and the courage to take new action in their personal lives" (p. 322). All of the women in Tisdale's study also expressed their efforts at grounding themselves spiritually as a way of creating "an integrated balance" (p. 324), which supported Pargament's supposition of the use of religion in maintaining a state of holistic well-being in marginalized groups. Pargament spoke of the impact of religion on the African-American community in terms of the church, while Tisdale discussed the influence of spirituality in learning environments—which explicitly included the church in the African-American culture. As poignantly expressed by Frazier (1964), "In providing a structured social life in which the Negro could give expression to his deepest feeling and at the same time achieve status and find a meaningful existence, the Negro church provided a refuge in a hostile white world" (p. 50). Thus, the African-American (Negro) church definitely served a myriad of needs in that community. In fact, Frazier portrays the Negro church as "a nation within a nation" in terms of its influences on social control, economic cooperation, education, and politics (pp.35-50).

Nye's (1993) investigation into the work of Frazier's (1964) research on the role of the church in African-American culture unveiled six salient subthemes affecting ways in which the African-American church functions:

1. An *expressive* function or an outlet for one's deepest emotions. This was found in the way in which many respondents couched their deepest concerns in religious terms and references;
2. A *status* function or religious participation confers recognition which may be lacking or denied in the wider, white-dominated world;
3. A *meaning* function or a source of order and understanding for one's life. This function is particularly important in maintaining continuity;
4. A *refuge* function as a haven in an oftentimes hostile world;
5. A *cathartic* function or as an avenue for the release of pent-up emotions and frustrations felt by an oppressed minority;
6. An *other worldly* orientation function, so named because it orients the person, self, and activities toward eventual fulfillment in the next life. This function is at least equal to the meaning function in maintaining continuity. (p. 105)

Boyd-Franklin and Lockwood (1999) added two additional functions to Nye's expansion of Frazier's work: social and child-rearing and socialization. These other two functions offer African-Americans the benefits of an extended family support system and socialization without acculturation:

7. A *social function,* that is, the opportunity to meet, socialize, and share fellowship with others who share a similar background and interests. This peer involvement can be especially important for adolescents vulnerable to pressures to join gangs, use drugs, or become sexually active.
8. A *child-rearing and socialization function,* which is especially important for single parents. Often churches provide baby-sitting during services in addition to the youth activities discussed above. (p. 95)

The overall depiction of Nye's and Boyd-Franklin and Lockwood's analysis of the African-American church was one of a safe haven—a place free of the dominant culture. In other words, it is a place where people's gifts can be recognized, where problems can be solved, and where there is hope (Walsh, 1999). A stern concept of reciprocity—mutual exchange, a process of giving and taking and sharing and receiving in community—seems to run through all eight of these functions. The use of the church as a safe haven has been especially true for African-American women. Various studies other studies (Billingsley & Caldwell, 1991; Mattis, 2002; Musgrave, Allen, & Allen, 2002) also supported the role of spirituality as the main source of coping for African-American women, suggesting that their very well-being is dependent on their relationships with God, the church, and each other. In fact, Isaac, Guy, and Valentine (2001) examined motivations of African-Americans' participation in church-based adult education and identified several factors: "(a) Familiar Cultural Setting, (b) Spiritual and Religious Development, (c) Love of Learning, (d) Support in Facing Personal Challenges, (e) Family Togetherness, (f) Service to Others, and (g) Social Interaction" (p. 27). These elements represent and support a transformative context for adult religious education, a context in which meaning-making, reflection, discernment, intuition, and transcendence work together in fostering transformative learning. There is a commonality among the various studies cited; they all recognized the significant role of religious involvement in our mental, social, and physical health (also see Levin, Chatters, & Taylor, 2005).

Research (Coe, 1919; Ellison, 1991) further supported a direct positive influence of religious involvement on well-being as a source of social integration. Ellison presented four major ways that religious involvement enhances the perception of well-being: social intercourse, social networks, social control, and meaning-making. Another study by Ellison and Gay (1990) targeted the effects of religion on African-Americans' well-being. However, this study did not focus on African-American women or the impact of participation on their coping abilities.

Musgrave, Allen, and Allen (2002, p. 557) conducted a study that contributed to the background of this research, which concluded that whether used separately or together, spirituality and religiosity alternate approach to coping. Research conducted by Musgrave et al. and Wiley, Warren, and Montanelli (2002) suggests participation in religious activities helps African-American women cope with the challenges of life. The use of prayer has been identified as a preferred religious activity used by African-Americans, especially women, as a coping mechanism (Ellison & Taylor, 1996; Mattis, 2002).

How, then, does participation in adult religious education affect the coping abilities of African-American women? Generally, an overall sense of well-being is the expected outcome of effective adult religious education or religious involvement (Ellison, 1990; Ellison, Boardman, Williams, & Jackson, 2001; Ellison & Gay, 1990; George, Ellison, & Larson, 2002). Several studies identify the impact of religious coping on well-being and the moderating effects related to negative events in various African-American populations (Brant & Pargament, 1995; Brown & Gary, 1988; Ellison, 1993; Ellison & Gay, 1990; Krause & Van Tran, 1989; O'Brien, 1982). Pargament (1997) found the following:

> Religious coping variables appear to be more consistently and more strongly related to outcomes than are general orientation variables. This pattern of results fits with the idea that religious coping acts as a mediator or bridge between general religious orientations and the outcomes of negative life events. (p. 286)

Although a review of the literature indicates a broad spectrum of approaches to the study of religion and coping, the focus of this current study will be from a transformative learning perspective (Mezirow, 1978, 1990, 1991, 2000). According to Mezirow, one's belief system is foundational to how one learns and makes sense of life experiences, especially traumatic situations or *disorienting dilemmas*.

Recognizing that not every traumatic situation may be considered a disorienting dilemma, the stress produced by a major life event and the accumulation of stress from everyday situations can be instrumental in perpetuating changes in the way one thinks and behaves (Wethington, 2003). While Mezirow acknowledges the gradual influence of life experiences as a cumulative trigger for cognitive and behavioral change, his approach to transformative adult learning identifies a disorienting dilemma as the starting point for perspective transformation.

While this current research embraces Mezirow's theory of perspective transformation as its theoretical framework, the presence of a disorienting dilemma is not presupposed. Considering the dynamics of adult religious education in the African-American church, it is likely that some participants would have experienced a disorienting dilemma.

▪ The Research Problem

A review of literature in the fields of learning, adult education, and adult religious education indicates a need for further culture and context specific studies that explore the relationship among these three areas. This present study begins the process of addressing such a need by exploring the impact of adult religious education on coping abilities of Protestant African-American women in southeast Mississippi. The need for this study is two-fold: (1) It will inform adult educators and healthcare providers of the importance of religion/spirituality in the lives of African-American women, and (2) It will inform decision-making all various levels—social, political, spiritual—when it comes to providing for the wellbeing of African-American women. Results from this study can contribute to the development of more inclusive mental health programs that involve various religious/spiritual aspects (e.g., prayer, meditation, spiritual retreat) can be developed to help African-American women cope with stressful events, which contributes to as overall state of health and wellbeing.

There is limited research in the area of African-American women and coping, from "both the psychology of religion and the psychology of women" (Mattis, 2002, p. 309) perspectives. However, Wiley et al. (2002) and Isaac et al. (2001) support the assumption that participation in church and religious activities is important to coping with stressful life events. Wiley et al. found that faith increased with church attendance, indicating a positive relationship (a reduction in stressful events) between parenting and religion among poor African-American mothers. How then, do African-American women (of any social status) cope with the exigent obligations facing them in the American society of the 21st century? It has been commonly expressed that African-Americans' participation in various religious or spiritual activities (e.g., worship, prayer, Bible study, mission, Sunday school, private prayer, meditation, etc.) helps them to cope with stress (Chatters, Levin, & Taylor, 1992; Levin, Taylor, & Chatters, 1994, 1995; Pargament, 1997). This anchoring in a higher power (God) as the key to African-Americans' well-being is supported by several studies that document a connection between well-being and religious involvement (Ellison, Boardman, Williams, Jackson, 2001; George, Ellison, & Larson, 2002; Krause, Ellison, & Marcum, 2002).

Although there were limited empirical data linking transformative learning with coping abilities in African-American women who participated regularly in religious activities, the researcher assumed a relationship existed because of the transformative power of religion and the dynamic nature of the African-American church. Mattis' (2002) study addressed this issue in terms of meaning-making and coping in church-based settings. A meta-analysis by Pargament (1997) examined religious coping in various settings with different populations, some of which included African-American women. Another study conducted by Mattis, Taylor, and Chatters (2001) supports the significance of religion for the well-being of African-American women in general, which provides a basis for more in-depth and broader studies on the relationship of religion as a coping resource for African-American women.

▪ Purpose of the Study and Research Questions

First, the general purpose of this study was to examine existing research on the topic of African-American women and coping to look for ways in which religious participation serves as perspective transformation, while influencing coping. Second, the study was designed to examine the effect of stressful life events and demographic variables on coping. Third, according to Mezirow and Associates (2000), various assumptions regarding transformative learning remain empirically unexplored as they relate to differences—"the role of class, culture, and ethnicity in the process of change, the role of context in shaping the transformative experience; and transformation as 'adult' learning theory" (pp. 287-288). Ultimately, this study took into consideration those uncharted territories of transformative learning identified by virtue of its target population: African-American women in African-American Protestant churches in southeast Mississippi.

African-American women are commonly known for their religiosity. Understanding that this religiosity is the source of African-American women's strength has implications for program planning on educational, religious, social, and psychological levels for the adult educator who seeks to reform and transform the socio-economic and political spheres of African-American women. Adult education and learning in the 21st century demand changes in how adult religious education is perceived, developed, and delivered. This current study will inform theory and practice in the area of transformative learning for adults in religious education that may have implications for other transformative learning environments involving African-American women who have a strong religious background.

> Taylor (1997) conducted an extensive overview of empirical studies that critiqued Mezirow's (1978, 1990, 1991) transformative learning theory. This current study—while not intended to serve as a critique—attempts to build upon Mezirow's transformative learning theory by expanding the concepts of critical reflection, context, and relationships. Although Taylor's extensive review of transformative learning research greatly informs the process of a perspective transformation, he admits that "only the surface has been scratched in understanding its nature and relationship to adult learning" (p. 51).

In conclusion, the specific purpose of this study on participation in adult religious education is to examine the impact of religious/spiritual involvement on Protestant African-American women's abilities to cope with stress—identifying activities and demographic factors that specifically influence coping strategies. The overarching premise was that adult religious education is a form of transformative learning that positively impacts African-American women's ability to cope with stressful life events.

The exploratory nature of the study—with transformative learning theory as a framework--allowed for the examination of the relationship between participation in adult religious education, the experience of stressful life events, and coping ability used a mixed method approach. The target population was Protestant African-American women in southeast Mississippi. Two research questions were addressed in this study: (1) How does the level of participation in adult religious education affect African-American women's coping abilities? (2) Is there a relationship between the experience of stressful life events, various demographics variables, and the choice of coping resources?

Definitions

The terms discussed in this study are very closely related. The inter-connectedness of the concepts and terms seemingly reflect the holistic nature of what it means to be human.

1. Adult religious education. Any organized participation in adult learning in a church-based or private setting where individuals explore religious/spiritual beliefs about God (e.g., worship service attendance, public prayer, Bible study, mission, Sunday school, vacation Bible school, conferences, seminars, retreats, special events, and other forms of religious training). A Christian orientation is used.
2. Discernment. "The quality of being able to grasp and comprehend what is obscure" (Mish et al., 1999, p. 330).
3. Health. "The general condition of the body or mind with reference to soundness and vigor" (Stein, Hauck, & Su, 1975, p. 609). The term will be used synonymously in this study with well-being to represent one's physiological, psychological, and spiritual condition as a whole (i.e., if the foot, head, or heart is sick, the whole body is sick).
4. Intuition. Mish et al. (1999) defined intuition as "an act of contemplating" and as "the power or faculty of attaining to direct knowledge or cognition without evident rational thought and inference" (p. 615).
5. Meaning perspectives/frame of reference. The two terms can be used interchangeably.

    [Meaning perspectives] are sets of meaning schemes that provide us with criteria for judging or evaluating right and wrong, bad and good, beautiful and ugly, true and false, appropriate and inappropriate. They also determine our concept of personhood, our idealized self-image, and the way we feel about ourselves (Mezirow, 1991, p. 44). In later research, "meaning perspectives" is replaced by the term "*frame of reference*," which means "habits of mind" and "resulting points of view" (Wiessner & Mezirow, 2000, p. 345).

6. Meaning schemes. Meaning schemes are sets of related and habitual expectations governing if-then, cause-effect, and category relationships as well as event sequences" (Mezirow, 1991, p. 2). The term "meaning schemes" was later defined as "elements constituting a point of view" derived from a new frame of reference (Wiessner & Mezirow, 2000, p. 345).
7. Religion. The private or corporate events or activities that lend themselves to an individual's spiritual growth (Pullen & Tuck, 1996). For the purpose of this study, religion/spirituality or

religious/spiritual will be used as one concept that represents the God presence or *practical transcendental activities and beliefs* inherent in learning in adult religious education.

8. Spiritual formation. "Christian spiritual formation is the process of being conformed to the image of Christ" (Mulholland, 1985, p. 27). Mulholland describes life as spiritual formation (p. 28), advocating that "Genuine spiritual formation brings about a radical shift from being our own production to being God's workmanship" (p. 29). Thus, the dynamics of life itself—when infused with religious/spiritual experiences—allow for changes in one's frame of reference that can lead to a perspective transformation. Life is a journey and spiritual formation is a process that allows Christians who engage it to find balance and wholeness.

9. Spirituality. The incomprehensible manner in which an individual relates to an internalized belief in a greater power (Pullen & Tuck, 1996). For the purpose of this study, spirituality will refer to anything the individual does to enhance her connectedness with God (e.g., meditation, private prayer, journal keeping, spiritual readings, dreams, visions, revelations, and any other experience deemed spiritual). As noted above, the term will be used in combination with religion (i.e., religion/spirituality, although two separate but related concepts, both represent an interdependent aspect of the transcendent).

10. Transcendent. Mish et al. (1999) defined transcendent as "exceeding usual limits" and "extending or lying beyond the limits of ordinary experience" (p. 1253). A second definition by Coyle (2002) that presents a dual approach to transcendence will also be used interchangeably with the definition offered by Mish et al.: "(a) *intrapersonal*, a type of inner knowledge of God; and (b) *transpersonal*, a connectedness with God based on *meaning* and *purpose* with other people" (p. 590).

11. Transformative Learning. Transformative learning is defined as follows:

> Transformative learning refers to the process by which we transform our taken-for-granted frames of references ... to make them more inclusive, discriminating, open, emotionally capable of change, and reflective so that they may generate beliefs and opinions that will prove more true or justified to guide action. (Mezirow, 2000, pp. 7-8)

12. Well-being. Well-being is defined as "a good or satisfactory condition of existence; a state characterized by health, happiness, and prosperity" (Stein et al., 1975, p. 1493). The term is used synonymously in this study with holistic health.

■ Limitations

This study targeted only African-American women in southeast Mississippi (predominantly the Hattiesburg-Pine Belt area) who were involved in Protestant church-based adult religious education and other personal spiritual disciplines (e.g., prayer, Bible reading, witnessing, and retreats). Therefore, the results of this research may not have broad generalizations for several reasons. First, this study is limited to Christian (primarily Protestant) women 21 years of age and over who are of African-American decent. Women of other ethnic, disenfranchised, or minority groups and men of any persuasion may not be affected spiritually and psychologically by the same factors that are true for African-American women.

Second, women of religious affiliations other than the Protestant faith may have varying degrees of differences (and similarities) in their view of spirituality and religious-based coping. It cannot be assumed that the source of strength related to religious practices for the women who participated in this study is related solely to the variables listed.

Third, the convenience sample for this study is taken from local churches within an extremely limited geographical region of the United States. The churches targeted are African-American Protestant congregations. Also, it cannot be assumed that non-affiliated women and women of other ethnic orientations from other geographical regions would not be strengthened primarily by their spirituality as well—realizing that spirituality is not limited to formalized denominational affiliation, Christian religious education, or traditional spiritual practices.

Fourth, the primary use of quantitative instruments in assessing subjective-based information limits interpretations to the rational and objective. However, religious/spiritual phenomena operate in the transcendent and subjective realms. The use of more qualitative data collection methods might benefit such a study.

▪ Justification

According to Tisdale (2001), "Until very recently, with the exception of adult *religious* education, spirituality has been given little attention in mainstream academic adult education" (p. 232), although several studies support spirituality as being a source of strength for disadvantaged groups (Hodge, 2001; Isaac et al., 2001; Musgrave et al., 2002; Schaller, 1996). Levin et al. (1996) identified several areas where religious affiliation impacted individual outcomes: "(a) sexual activity, (b) criminal behavior, contraceptive usage, (c) social support, (d) fertility, (e) marital happiness, (f) attitudes toward the environment, (g) and even reports of paranormal experiences" (p. 220). According to Tisdale (2001), "Given the connection between adult learning and adult development, discussions of spiritual development are relevant to concerns in adult education" (p. 232). The insight offered by Tisdale clearly indicates a need for a more culturally relevant approach to adult learning that is both inclusive and emancipatory (p. 233).

Thus, this study addressed adult learning from a religious/spiritual context, providing grounds for the practical application of a holistic approach to health and empowerment of African-American women—who have suffered at the hands of racial, gender, economic, political, and social injustices since the slavery of the African people in America (Brant & Pargament, 1995; DuBois, 1989). In some sense, adult religious education was seen as emancipatory, as indicated by Tisdale's (2000) study:

> In fact, the study suggests that spiritual development appears to require a rational component; it is important to critically think about one's spiritual experience not as a substitute for the spiritual experience itself, but because critically analyzing messages from the larger culture, including one's religion, is an important part of claiming one's own identity. (pp. 332-333)

Although the abolishment of destructive social systems may not be realistic and may not level the playing field, results from this current study will better equip adult educators, adult religious educators, and healthcare professionals to facilitate transformative learning environments—environments essential for African-American women's well-being.

CHAPTER II
LITERATURE REVIEW

▓ Introduction

This chapter presents an overview of the transformative theory, two case studies from the Bible as examples of perspective transformation, and a discussion of key elements related to transformative learning. Background information on several topics is offered: (a) the role of religion/spirituality on health, (b) stress and coping, (c) adult religious education and learning, (d) religious education, (e) philosophies and theories of religious education, (f) philosophies of adult education, and (g) theories of adult learning.

▓ Transformation Theory

The transformation theory, according to Mezirow (1991), "seeks to explain the way adult learning is structured and to determine by what processes the frames of reference through which we view and interpret our experience (meaning perspectives) are changed or transformed" (p. xiii). This study engages the transformative learning process from a spiritual dimension—adult religious education. How do one's religious/spiritual experiences contribute to a change in perspective or transformation? Is one changed or formed spiritually because of some disruptive life crisis? How does one's belief in God help one cope with disorienting dilemmas? To explore these questions, we must understand what is involved in the transformative learning process.

▓ *Transformative Learning*

Transformative learning demands a critical evaluation of one's life scripts. What we believe must be challenged and re-challenged through intentional reflection in an effort to understand why we feel, believe, and react the way we do to environmental stimuli (Mezirow 1990, p. 18). According to Mezirow (2000),

> A defining condition of being human is our urgent need to understand and order the meaning of our experience, to integrate it with what we know to avoid the threat of chaos. If we are unable to understand, we often turn to tradition, thoughtlessly seize explanations by authority figures, or resort to various psychological mechanisms, such as projection and rationalization, to create imaginary meanings. (p. 3)

9

Transformative learning lays life's experiences under the microscope of reflective criticism in an effort to create a sense of balance—a way of making peace with one's self. Thus, the repertoire of life experiences embedded in chaotic situations creates an environment ripe for transformative learning by means of a reflective process that ultimately leads to acquiring skills essential to meaning-making.

Inevitably, experience can be rated by virtue of its context. Biblical text read out of context—without an understanding of its setting—puts one at risk for "isogesis" rather than exegesis. Clearly, a scripture out of context takes on a meaning not intended by the original writer. So it is with adult learning. When one cannot make sense of one's experiences, those experiences are rendered almost meaningless—or one is left confused and with the wrong meaning. The meaning-making of transformative learning appropriates the meaning needed to write new life scripts from old contexts—socially, culturally, politically, and spiritually. How we assimilate and manage the new knowledge gained from these meaningful experiences comes because of critical reflection—which is decisive to the transformative learning process. Mezirow (1990) states, "While all reflection implies an element of critique, the term *critical reflection* will here be reserved to refer to challenging the validity of *presuppositions* in prior learning" (p. 12). According to Mezirow (2000),

> Transformative learning refers to the process by which we transform our taken-for-granted frames of references (meaning perspectives, habits of mind, mind-sets) to make them more inclusive, discriminating, open, emotionally capable of change, and reflective so that they may generate beliefs and opinions that will prove more true or justified to guide action. Transformative learning involves participation in constructive discourse to use the experience of others to assess reasons justifying these assumptions, and making an action decision based on the resulting insights. (pp. 8-9)

Mezirow (2000) argues that there are four different ways transformative learning can occur: (a) by elaborating existing frames of reference, (b) by learning new frames of reference, (c) by transforming points of view, and (d) by transforming habits of mind (p. 19). The transformation process demands that the learner be an active participant in re-establishing the scheme of his or her life—questioning whatever does not fit the relevant *frame of reference*. Critical reflection is essential to this entire meaning-making process. It would be a challenge to make valid associations to a *frame of reference* without engaging critical and reflective thinking. The learner must relate to the inner person in order to fully understand the new direction he or she is taking. Transformative learning demands change.

Transformative learning is essential to the human situation. This theory is grounded in and reflective of change. The adult learner grows and changes everyday. Each life circumstance lends itself to the opportunity to learn and to make changes that may lead to transformation. The transformation may be intentional or it may be subtle or accidental; nonetheless, the power of change will affect the human life. The extent of change may depend on the depth of the crisis that leads to that change. Mezirow's theory supports the idea that one of the tasks of the adult educator is to help facilitate an understanding of the transformative learning process, promoting the assimilation and application of new learning.

▦ *Perspective Transformation*

The reflective and meaning-making components of transformative learning aid the adult learner in taking life's experiences under consideration at various times in order to make sense of the moment. According to Mezirow (1991),

> [Perspective transformation is] the process of becoming critically aware of how and why our assumptions have come to constrain the way we perceive, understand, and feel about our world; changing these structures of habitual expectation to make possible a more inclusive, discriminating, and integrative perspective; and finally, making choices or otherwise acting upon these new understandings. (p. 167)

What we know, believe, and value is connected to the context of our lives in those defining moments—socially, politically, and spiritually. Participants in Tisdale's (2000) study indicated that "what was described as significant spiritual experiences did result in the courage to take new action first in their personal lives" (p. 331). The meaning-making of transformative learning appropriates value to new experiences based on the integration of new knowledge with old knowledge to yield perspective transformation. The stages of perspective transformation, although not necessarily linear, indicate how the appropriation and re-appropriation of knowledge as a result of significant life experiences may ultimately lead to lifestyle changes.

Stages of perspective transformation. Mezirow's (1978, 1991) perspective transformation theory—which is the conceptual framework for this study—suggests the presence of a *disorienting dilemma* as the basis for transformation. However, the present research does not assume the presence of a single triggering factor; rather, an accumulation of triggers over time is presumed—not barring the possibility of a single disorienting event. The following is a list of the ten stages Mezirow (1991) identified in his theory of perspective transformation:

1. A disorienting dilemma
2. Self-examination with feelings of guilt or shame
3. A critical assessment of epistemic, sociocultural, or psychic assumptions
4. Recognition that one's discontent and the process of transformation are shared and that others have negotiated a similar change
5. Exploration of options for new roles, relationships, and actions
6. Planning a course of action
7. Acquisition of knowledge and skills for implementing one's plans
8. Provisional trying of new roles
9. Building of competence and self-confidence in new roles and relationships; and
10. A reintegration into one's life on the basis of conditions dictated by one's new perspective. (pp. 168-169)

Saint Paul's disorienting dilemma. According to Mezirow (1990), "Perspective transformation occurs in response to an externally imposed disorienting dilemma—a divorce, death of a loved one, change in job status, retirement, or other" (pp. 13-14). The story of Saint Paul is told in the book of

Acts. Paul (then called Saul) was going about his routine task of persecuting Christians when a light appeared from heaven and a voice called out to him as he traveled on the Damascus Road:

> And he fell to the earth, and heard a voice saying unto him, Saul, Saul, why persecutest thou me?
>
> And he said, Who art thou, Lord? And the Lord said, I am Jesus whom thou persecutest: it is hard for thee to kick against the pricks.
>
> And he trembling and astonished said, Lord, what wilt thou have me to do? And the Lord said unto him, Arise, and go into the city, and it shall be told thee what thou must do.
>
> And the men which journeyed with him stood speechless, hearing a voice, but seeing no man.
>
> And Saul arose from the earth; and when his eyes were opened, he saw no man: but they led him by the hand, and brought him into Damascus.
>
> And he was three days without sight, and neither did eat nor drink. (Acts 9:4-9)

Saint Paul's Damascus Road conversion certainly qualifies as a unique religious experience and a disorienting dilemma—typifying a perspective transformation:

- Step 1. The sudden fall from his horse and the experience that followed was disconcerting, a disorienting dilemma (Acts 9:1-4).
- Step 2. The personal encounter with Jesus caused him to examine personal feelings of guilt and shame (Acts 9:5).
- Step 3. He certainly must have critically reevaluated his previously held assumptions about Christianity (Acts 9:6-8).
- Step 4. There was a realization that there were many others who had become discontented with their previous beliefs and had been converted to Christianity (Acts 9:9-12).
- Step 5. Saint Paul must have recognized that with his conversion, there would inevitably be a new allegiance with new roles and relationships (Acts 9:13-14).
- Step 6. A change in perspective leads to a change in course of action. The change in this instance was very dramatic. Saint Paul became the savior of the very people he had been persecuting (Acts 9:15-16).
- Step 7. His visit from Ananias began his journey to new knowledge and skills for the task ahead (Acts 9:17-18).
- Step 8. Saint Paul began preaching the gospel of Jesus Christ (Acts 9:19-21).
- Step 9. His confidence in his conversion and new role as preacher increased with his proclamation of the gospel (Acts 9:22-25).
- Step 10. Saint Paul's visit with other believers and the powerful preaching ministry that followed validated his acceptance and integration of his changed perspective on life (Acts 9:26-31).

Mezirow's (1978, 1991) stages of perspective transformation are exemplified in Paul's conversion experience and subsequent ministry. Paul experienced a complete turn around in his life. The perspective transformation exemplary of Saint Paul's conversion experience qualifies as a disorienting dilemma. As extraordinary as some experiences are, the gradual transformations that occur as an accumulation of daily living (and through the lifelong process of adult religious education) are still products of transformative learning. The biblical examples offered in the next section are indicative of gradual changes in meaning perspectives, which may be more representative of Boyd and Myers' (1988) discernment approach to transformation. The discernment perspective on transformation suggests a greater reliance on the transcendent or supernatural in making-meaning and managing life's daily affairs. Mezirow (1991) reported that his phases of perspective transformation were confirmed in the work of Morgan (1987). Morgan indicated, "Women often turned to religion for solace after experiencing the guilt and shame of critical self-reflection" (p. 169). Morgan's research supports the importance of the role of religion/spirituality in meaning-making.

Meaning-making. Taylor (1997) is of the opinion that the studies reviewed in his critique of Mezirow validate the reality of perspective transformation gained from various adult life experiences. A study conducted by Courtenay, Merriam, and Reeves (1996), examined the way in which personal illness acts as a catalyst for meaning-making upon receiving a life-threatening diagnosis. Such a diagnosis could be considered a disorienting dilemma. Courtenay et al. (1996) state, "The catalytic event appears to move individuals toward a concern for making meaning of their dilemma" (p. 78). Courtenay et al. propose an internal or external event that causes the learner to challenge old assumptions, motivating them to take some type of action as they try to make sense of their HIV-positive diagnosis. According to Courtenay et al.,

> The initial reaction period is that time when the self attempts to draw from the old assumptions to explain the disorienting dilemma; it is critical to the meaning-making process because for transformation to occur, the individual must recognize that the old assumptions are inadequate for making sense of the present dilemma. (p. 78)

Courtenay et al. identified three phases in their meaning-making theory: "(a) Phase I, exploration and experimentation; (b) Phase II, consolidation of new meaning; and (c) Phase III, stabilization of new perspective" (pp. 72-76). These three phases are comparable to Mezirow's (1991) finding that "Perspective transformation involves (a) an empowered sense of self, (b) more critical understanding of how one's social relationships and culture have shaped one's beliefs and feelings, and (c) more functional strategies and resources for taking action" (p. 161). Both models require the type of critical reflection essential for transformative meaning-making.

More specifically, Courtenay et al.'s first phase calls into question the nuts and bolts of problem-solving. "In this first phase of the meaning-making process, respondents paused to take stock of their identity and their purpose for being here. Old views of life were challenged and new perceptions about life and their roles in it began to emerge" (p. 74). This concept resembles what happens to the non-believer once he or she accepts Jesus Christ as Lord and Savior. The adult religious education experience nurtures believers as they engage the challenges of this new journey—which serves as a meaning-making process that continues throughout the adult lifespan.

Phase II is characterized by the cognitive processes involved in the previous stage (Courtenay et al., 1996, pp. 74-75). Phase III, which builds on Phase I and Phase II, produces an assimilation of "new perceptions and articulates the meaning of having a life-threatening disease." This continuous process of critical reflection and meaning-making supports the tenets of Mezirow's (1991) perspective transformation theory.

When the balance of mind, body, and soul is unstable, there is a resulting disequilibrium (Doctor & Doctor, 1994; Gehrels, 1984). Whether internally or externally produced, the sense of being out of control causes one to search for ways of bringing everything back into perspective. It is feasible to think that the way in which this re-balancing of the self takes place depends largely on one's environment.

Discernment of the transcendent. Although a criticism of Mezirow's theory is that it appears weak on the spiritual dimension, Mezirow (1991), while not addressing the issue directly, did allude to the transcendent in his reference to "unconscious dimensions" According to Mezirow, "Perspective transformation often involves profound changes in self, changes with cognitive, emotional, somatic, and unconscious dimensions" (p. 177). Situations in adult religious education settings that lend themselves to these types of changes—though unconscious—can expect to be transcendent in nature.

In this current study, spirituality is viewed as a means of discerning the unconscious or the transcendent dimension. Perhaps the search for meaning is internally motivated by the soul's desire to know God better as life experiences awaken the soul's stirrings to a God-consciousness, a consciousness that results when the Holy Spirit embodies the soul. Perhaps the Christian's transformative learning results when the mind, body, and soul begin to make sense of the spiritual things of God. Saint Paul writes, "That ye may approve things that are excellent; that ye may be sincere and without offence till the day of Christ" (Philippians 1:10). Discernment is a way of understanding from a spiritual perspective. Elias (1997) concluded the following:

> While Mezirow argues that transformative learning only happens through critical analysis of underlying premises, Jungians argue that a worldview is shaped not only by the rational assumptions in the personal unconscious, but by the symbolic meaning, through the direct apprehension and appropriation of frameworks of meaning that emerge freshly from the unconscious. This process is described as discernment, an appreciative and receptive process that stands in sharp contrast with Mezirow's emphasis on critical reflection. (p. 3)

Saint James presents discernment in terms of wisdom: "If any of you lack wisdom, let him ask of God, that giveth to all men liberally, and upbraideth not; and it shall be given him" (James 1:5). Wisdom is a practical approach to discernment, a way of applying understanding to situations. The write of this following pericope assumed his listeners understood more than they really did—that they possessed discernment.

> Of whom we have many things to say, and hard to be uttered, seeing ye are dull of hearing.
> For when for the time ye ought to be teachers, ye have need that one teach you again which be the first principles of the oracles of God; and are become such as have need of milk, and not of strong meat.
> For every one that useth milk is unskilful in the word of righteousness: for he is a babe.
> But strong meat belongeth to them that are of full age, even those who by reason of use have their senses exercised to discern both good and evil. (Hebrews 5:11-14)

Jewish Christians were hesitant to change their old *frame of reference* regarding religious doctrines. They were now face to face with the teachings of Jesus, the great High Priest (Hebrews 4:14-5:10, New Living Translation). The Jewish Christians' lack of maturity can be associated with their inability to critically reflect on the new teachings of Jesus and their failure to discern his true identity as High Priest.

> Our capacity to feast on deeper knowledge of God ("solid food") is determined by our spiritual growth. Too often we want God's banquet before we are spiritually capable of digesting it. As you grow in the Lord and put into practice what you have learned, your capacity to understand will also grow. (*Life Application Study Bible* [LASB], 1996, p. 1967)

Throughout these biblical passages, references were made to learning that indicated a change in how one interprets and applies knowledge. It can be argued, then, that adult religious education has the catalytic capacity to deepen one's total awareness of the transcendent—expanding the capacity for critical reflection and discernment. This research explored the concepts of discernment and transcendence as elements of transformative learning. African-American women's reliance on religion/spirituality is explored as a means of coping, with consideration for the roles of discernment, critical reflection, and meaning-making in the transformative learning process. The role of relationship is also critical to transformative learning, particularly as it relates to community—relationship with God and each other (Belenky, Clinchy, Goldberger, & Tarule, 1986).

Thus, another way of knowing within the context of this study was that of divine origin—transcendent and intuitive. Spirituality implies a different way of knowing that transcends human understanding. In the religious context, critical reflection could easily be viewed as meditation or contemplation. Foster (1998) defines meditation as "listening to God's word, reflecting on God's works, rehearsing God's deeds, ruminating on God's law, and more" (p. 15). For African-American women, the church becomes the context—the classroom—for learning that changes or transforms her old ways of knowing. Her outlook on life is often affected by the teachings and relationships she is exposed to in her religious environment. The way she experiences God is thought to play a major role in the way she copes with stress. Her participation in religious education activities is considered essential to her well-being as she assimilates new information and re-negotiates purpose.

Frame of reference and the adult learner. Assimilating information and negotiating purpose is fundamental to the transformative learning process. This assimilation process is crucial if adult learners are to play an active role in creating new meaning out of their life experiences. Mezirow's (2000) constructivist viewpoint proposes four different ways for this transformative learning to occur: (a) by elaborating existing frames of reference, (b) by learning new frames of reference, (c) by transforming points of view, and (d) by transforming habits of mind (p. 19). The process of transformation demands that the learner be an active participant in re-establishing the scheme of his or her life—questioning whatever does not fit the relevant frame of reference. Critical reflection is essential to this entire meaning-making process.

Valid associations cannot be made for any frame of reference without engaging critical and reflective thinking. The learner must relate to the inner person in order to fully understand the new direction he or she is taking. Transformative learning demands change—change that result from critical reflection and all that goes into the meaning-making process. The application of new insight and understanding that is derived from a different "frame of reference" serves to empower the adult learner to move in the direction of positive change. Dworkin (1959) details Dewey's *pedagogic creed* that begins with a descriptive definition of education:

> I believe that all education proceeds by the participation of the individual in the social consciousness of the race. This process begins unconsciously almost at birth, and is continually shaping the individual's powers, saturating his consciousness, forming his habits, training his ideas, and arousing his feelings and emotions. (p. 19)

Baumgartner (2002) described learning and development as inseparable and lifelong, stating succinctly: "Learning continuously reshapes people" (p. 44). Thus, each life circumstance and challenge can be seen as an opportunity to learn, to change, and to be transformed. Transformation may be unintentional or it may be subtle or accidental. Nonetheless, the power of change will affect the human life. The extent depends on the depth of the crisis that leads to the change.

Wiessner and Mezirow (2000) suggest that the role of the adult educator in this process is one of "co-learner" (p. 340). Perhaps as co-learner the adult educator is better able to facilitate an understanding of the transformative learning process, helping the learner assimilate and apply new knowledge through critical reflection.

A proposition of this study is that the acquisition and application of this new knowledge serves to empower the adult learner to move in the direction of positive change as a result of transformative learning in the same way that participation in adult religious education motivates critical reflection and strengthens coping abilities in African-American women. Belenky and Staton (2000) support the premise that Mezirow's transformation theory itself is a coping strategy that allows for critical reflection (p. 72). While Baumgartner (2002) considers critical reflection the "lynchpin" (p. 46) of transformative learning, one of the criticisms of transformation theory is its failure to incorporate the emotional aspect of learning (Wiessner & Mezirow, 2000). Wiessner and Mezirow depict intuition as an aspect of emotion, with intuition described as a way of reflecting and knowing that promotes transformative learning (p. 335).

Dewey (1933) presents an extensive discourse on the process of thinking that places reflection at the core of cognitive processes as he attempts to define "thinking." Dewey makes the following comment:

> Reflection involves not simply a sequence of ideas, but a *con-sequence*—a consecutive ordering in such a way that each determines the next as its proper outcome, while each outcome in turn leans back on, or refers to, its predecessors. The successive portions of a reflective thought grow out of one another and support one another; they do not come and go in a medley. Each phase is a step from something to something—technically speaking, it is a *term* of thought. Each term leaves a deposit that is utilized in the next term. The stream or flow becomes a train or chain. (pp. 5-6)

Dewey sees reflection as a progressive and valuable process that suggests belief and meaning. From Dewey's (1933) perspective, reflective thinking is critical to meaning-making in that each thought builds upon another with some end result in mind. Dewey suggests "no lines of demarcation" between the various operations that comprise the thinking process (p. 9). Perhaps this notion of "no lines of demarcation" might very well apply to the critical reflection, intuition, and discernments as elements of transformative learning.

Taylor (2000) proposed an interdependent relationship between critical reflection and affective learning, which supports a premise of this current study that the very nature of adult religious education demands affective learning. Therefore, the roles of intuition and discernment in religion/ spirituality are critical to coping and well-being.

▓ Stress and Coping

Zamble and Gekoski (1994) perceive coping as a way of responding to stressful situations, thus stress and coping are always linked (p. 1). Zamble and Gekoski expound on the theory of stress and coping developed by Lazarus and Folkman (1984) in relation to appraisal, which has primary and secondary functions in the coping process:

1. Primary [appraisal] entails an individual evaluating a situation as taxing resources and potentially problematic for his or her well-being.
2. In secondary appraisal, possible courses of action are generated and assessed as to how effectively they can meet the demand and thereby reduce the threat of well-being; in the process, one or more strategies are selected. (p. 3)

▓ *Assessment of Stress*

Doctor and Doctor (1994) report, "Other researchers have proposed that the stress response is mediated by covert or overt cognitive appraisal of events impinging on the individual that interprets these events as either threatening or not, and concomitantly assesses the individual's ability to handle the stressor" (p. 311). The processing—conscious or unconscious—of the threat of events to one's well-being demands a physiological and psychological response (Cohen, Kessler, & Gordon, 1995; Doctor & Doctor, 1994; Lazarus & Folkman, 1984; Zamble & Gekoski, 1994). And in view of the religious aspect of coping in this present study, one might add a spiritual response to the repertoire of coping resources. In fact, Mattis (2002) argues that "the most consistent findings regarding the coping experiences of African-American women are that religion and spirituality hold central places in these women's coping repertoires" (p. 309).

Prayer as a coping strategy. Prayer as the major coping strategy mentioned or alluded to by examples presented in this study, although not totally an unconscious act, might occur involuntarily as a natural response to stressful situations. After a particularly stressful incident one might say, "Lord, have mercy, Jesus!" Needless to say, the dynamic nature of the appraisal-based approach to coping requires the effective use of adequate coping resources. Zamble & Gekoski (1994) suggest "a certain level of health or energy, certain positive beliefs, problem-solving skills, social skills, social support, material resources, etc." (p. 3). The spontaneous prayer, "Lord, have mercy, Jesus!" possibly involves energy and the positive belief that God hears and answers prayer.

Doctor and Doctor (1994) suggest that primary appraisal identifies the threat generated from the stressful situation while secondary appraisal assigns the stressor associated with the threat (p. 314). However, Doctor and Doctor take the process one step further than Zamble and Gekoski (1994) by adding a third stage—coping responses, which are described in terms of an adaptive continuum. The five coping strategies they identified in relation to this process were "[1] seeking information, [2] direct action toward the situation, [3] inhibition of inappropriate emotional or behavioral reactions, [4] intrapsychic efforts to deal with feelings and negative beliefs, and [5] turning to others to work with feelings, gain support, and so on" (p. 314). The examples used in this study about Hagar of the Old Testament and Harriet Tubman presented two women who faced extraordinary challenges that required them to employ essential coping resources and strategies. Assuming these women's coping abilities were taxed to the limit because of inadequate or depleted resources, presumably, they turned to God as their primary source.

Hagar's hurdle. Hagar, the slave of Sarai, was asked by her mistress to bare a child by her husband, Abram, so that the promise of God for Abram to become the father of many nations might be fulfilled. According to Old Testament records:

> Now Sarai Abram's wife bare him no children: and she had an handmaid, an Egyptian, whose name was Hagar.
>
> And Sarai said unto Abram, Behold now, the Lord hath restrained me from bearing: I pray thee, go in unto my maid; it may be that I may obtain children by her. And Abram hearkened to the voice of Sarai.
>
> And Sarai Abram's wife took Hagar her maid the Egyptian, after Abram had dwelt ten years in the land of Canaan, and gave her to her husband Abram to be his wife.
>
> And he went in unto Hagar, and she conceived: and when she saw that she had conceived, her mistress was despised in her eyes.
>
> And Sarai said unto Abram, My wrong be upon thee: I have given my maid into thy bosom; and when she saw that she had conceived, I was despised in her eyes: the Lord judge between me and thee. (Genesis 16:1-5)

In this pericope, Sarai, the slave owner, has asked Hagar to be a surrogate mother for her. Since Hagar is a slave, she has no power of her own—not even over her own body. No external coping resources were available to her. Hagar did not so much as have the option of refusing her mistress. Sarai failed to understand the magnitude of her demand on her handmaiden. Hagar was asked to have sexual relations with Abram until she was pregnant, after which, she was to carry this child for nine months and then hand him over to Sarai. Something feels very cold about the situation that Hagar has been forced into. Perhaps the religious dimension of coping is all that is left (external locus of control), assuming Hagar had resigned to hopelessness.

Imagine the pain and conflict (the anger) that Hagar might have been internalizing toward Sarai and Abram? Hagar was forced to share intimacy with a man and to bear his child and then let both the man and the child go. Was Hagar expected not to love the man or the child? If there ever has been a disorienting dilemma, this situation definitely qualifies. In the verses that follow, Abram passes the buck back to Sarai:

> But Abram said unto Sarai, Behold, thy maid is in thine hand; do to her as it pleaseth thee. And when Sarai dealt hardly with her, she fled from her face.

And the angel of the LORD found her by a fountain of water in the wilderness, by the fountain in the way to Shur.

And he said, Hagar, Sarai's maid, whence camest thou? and whither wilt thou go? And she said, I flee from the face of my mistress Sarai.

And the angel of the LORD said unto her, Return to thy mistress, and submit thyself under her hands.

And the angel of the LORD said unto her, I will multiply thy seed exceedingly, that it shall not be numbered for multitude.

And the angel of the LORD said unto her, Behold, thou art with child and shalt bear a son, and shalt call his name Ishmael; because the LORD hath heard thy affliction. (Genesis 16:6-11)

The biblical text does not give a record of Hagar praying. Thus, three things might be assumed here: (a) Hagar prayed and it was not recorded, (b) she prayed silently, or (c) the Lord interceded on Hagar's behalf. How the Lord got involved in Hagar's situation is not certain. However, the fact remains: Hagar's help came from God. Her situation loomed larger than life and she had nowhere to turn. Her response to the angel's command reflects a spirit of faith and obedience. Hagar undoubtedly trusted God to take care of her in her situation and to fulfill the promise that was revealed by the angel. Hagar's hope was in the promise. If nothing else, the promise of a prosperous future enabled Hagar to cope with her current circumstance. Hagar is one of many biblical witnesses whose life testifies to the power of God to transform human conditions. For Hagar to cope, to manage her stressful situation, without physical resources would require her to depend solely on psychological and spiritual responses. Lazarus and Folkman (1984) defined coping as "constantly changing cognitive and behavioral efforts to manage specific external and/or internal demands that are considered taxing or exceeding the resources of the person" (p. 141). For sure, Hagar's situation far exceeded her resources.

Harriet's dilemma. Harriet Tubman is another example of extreme stress. Her victimization during American slavery in the 1800s was not much different from Hagar's Egyptian enslavement during ancient Bible times, requiring extraordinary coping abilities. Like Hagar, Harriet had to turn to God to see her through the bitter circumstances of her life that were precipitated by the institution of slavery. Taylor (1990) sums up Harriet's accomplishments rather neatly in the following passage:

Tubman escaped from slavery in 1849, and then returned to the South at least 19 times during the next 10 years to lead more than 300 Blacks to freedom in the North. According to one historian, No fugitive was ever captured who had [her] for a leader.' (p. 11)

This succinctly stated summation of Harriet's triumphs does not begin to represent the terrors involved in such a heroic life. Given the racial climate during the early 19th century, one can only imagine the life and death situations Harriet must have encountered almost daily as a result of her antislavery activities.

What happened in Harriet's life to cause this radical change? Was there a disorienting dilemma that perpetuated her move from slave to activist? According to Taylor,

> By the time she was 13, Harriet Ross [later Tubman] had seen sisters, brothers, and friends sold "down the river" to work on the vast cotton and sugar plantations of the Deep South.
>
> The childhood of a slave was short. When Harriet was five years old, her master rented her to a local couple named Cook. At their home, the little girl slept on the kitchen floor, poking her feet under the fireplace ashes when the nights grew cold. For meals, she shared table scraps with the Cook's dogs. (p. 21)

This excerpt is but a glimpse into the horrific nightmare that characterized Harriet's life (and probably the lives of every slave woman in America prior to their emancipation). According to Taylor (1990), in another gruesome experience it is reported that Harriet received a head wound that—had it been medically diagnosed—might have been identified as "a fractured skull and severe concussion" (p. 24). How had she survived this and the many other injustices common to slave women? Taylor states,

> Harriet had inherited her parents' strong religious faith, and as she slowly recovered from her head wound, she prayed hard—for the soul of plantation owner Edward Brodas. Years later, she told her first biographer, Sarah Bradford, about these days. 'As I lay so sick on my bed, from Christmas til March, I was always praying for old master,' she said. 'Oh, dear Lord,' she begged, 'change that man's heart and make him a Christian.' Although Brodas kept sending possible purchasers to look at her, she kept praying for him. 'All I could say,' she recalled, was, 'Oh, Lord, convert old master.' (pp. 25-26)

Conceivably there were many disconcerting circumstances in Harriet's life. It is likely that the culmination of these events eventually led her to become an activist. Regardless, Harriet's faith in God was obvious because of her diligent praying, which was clearly one of her chief means of coping. The vital role spirituality played as a coping strategy for women of color in ancient history and during slavery continues to be just as valuable for modern-day African-American women. A chronicle of women throughout history would reveal that the fate of African-American women has long been weighed by faith—trust and dependence on God.

Although this study does not chronicle the plight of African-American women through the ages, it does attempt to present the reader with a general picture of abuse and discrimination consistent with the oppression of minority groups and the role of religion/spirituality in coping with stress. DuBois (1989) resonates with the struggle when he writes:

> One ever feels his twoness—an American, a Negro; two souls, two thoughts, two unreconciled strivings; two warring ideals in one dark body, whose dogged strength alone keeps it from being torn asunder.
>
> The history of the American Negro is the history of this strife—this longing to attain self-conscious manhood, to merge his double self into a better and truer self. In this merging, he wishes neither of the older selves to be lost. He would not Africanize America, for America has too much to teach the world and Africa. (p.3)

The word of God has been used in worship, study, and prayer to aid in the reconciliation alluded to in this passage. The religious/spiritual life helps de-program old carnal ways of thinking and reprogram Christians for participation in a new way of life that is inherently transcendent. Historically, religious and spiritual convictions have been of vital importance in helping African-American women make sense of their world (Mattis, 2002).

■ *African-American Women and Meaning-making*

African-American women are often challenged with the task of managing with scarce or depleted social and material resources (Musgrave et al., 2002; Walsh, 1999). Walsh highlights the strong connection between African-American families who move away from home and their need to quickly find another church. According to Boyd-Franklin and Lockwood, (1999), "This connection may be extremely important for African-American clients isolated from natural support systems" (p. 94). What role, then, does religion/spirituality play in African-American women's ability to cope with stressful life events? To what do they owe their tenacious coping abilities? As supported by the literature reviewed in this study, the reliance on prayer and faith in God at such challenging times has been a primary coping resource for African-American women who are accustomed to using whatever is left to pull together a meal, a marriage, or any other matter at hand.

Commitments. It is premised in this current study that African-American women's belief in and commitment to God as evidenced by their participation in adult religious education and private spiritual disciplines strengthens coping abilities. Commitments are not only spiritual but also communal; they encompass one's total personal and social being: commitment to self, family, friends, school, work, and recreation. For this study, commitments also include the relationships that are based on the parishioner's relationship with the church. Zamble and Gekoski (1994) argue that the dynamics of the appraisal process discussed here are based on commitments and beliefs:

> Commitments refer to those things that are important to the individual, and thus include such things as values, other people, and activities to which a person may feel committed. Beliefs refer to the expectations that individual has regarding how the world in which he or she lives operates. (p. 3)

The interactive nature of evaluating and assessing beliefs and actions in appraisal coping resonates with the critical reflection component of perspective transformation.

Relationships. Relationships are also considered essential to the meaning-making process. Throughout life, adults are constantly engaged in different kinds of relationships.

According to Pargament (1998), the importance of relationships in meaning-making is reflected in his statement that "Relationships are another set of mechanisms in the search of significance" (p. 42). Belenky et al. (1998) postulated a theory of knowing specific to women that suggests a gender-related inequality that complicates the problem of finding one's voice in various relationships.

Since 1995, my practice in ministry has been focused on the spiritual formation of African-American women. This spiritual formation was always centered on small group activities (e.g., Bible study, prayer meetings, fellowship, outreach, retreats, seminars, and workshops) that involved other women. In these various small group settings, women found themselves in a myriad of relationships that proved foundational to their entire transformational experience. In fact, the very nature of adult religious education is grounded in transformational learning and relationships.

Groome (1980) states, "Religious education focuses specific attention on empowering people in their quest for a transcendent and ultimate ground of being. It leads people to consciousness of what is found, relationship with it, and expression of that relationship" (p. 22). The majority of the parishioners in worship services on Sunday morning in African-American churches are usually women—women who are involved in relationships with God, men, children, and each other. It might be reasonable to assert that relationships partially determine how women make sense of their environment (Achterberg, 1998; Ettling & Hayes, 1997). Sarai and Hagar were each in relationship with God, Abraham, Isaac, Ishmael, and the people of their village. Harriet Tubman was in relationship with her various masters, her family, and the emancipators who helped her to freedom. For Christians, their relationships with God is just as—if not more—essential as it other types of relationships.

■ *Philosophies and Theories of Religious Education, Adult Education, and Learning*

According to Elkins (1999), "Spirituality is the fastest growing—one of the only growing—sector of the publishing industry, with literally millions buying books on the theme" (para. 9). This driving thirst for intimacy with God indicates that something is missing in people's lives. A review of the literature identified a need for sociological, physiological, and psychological well-being (Fontana, 2003; Leach, 1957; McCann, 1962; Pargament, 1997). Therefore, any attempt to discuss adult religious education apart from adult education and culture would be incomplete. Religious beliefs are intricately linked to who we are, where we are, where we come from, and where we are going. Any discussion of religion/spirituality apart from the cultural and socio-political contexts would present false dichotomies (Groome, 1980, p. 26).

Elias (1993) provides a full discussion of the relationship between adult education and adult religious education. Groome (1980) purports, "The term *religious education* accurately describes the general investigation of the religious dimension of life and the common human quest for a transcendent ground of being" (p. 24). Groome sees religious education as a community affair that introduces a relationship between religious traditions and the transcendent (p. 24). Groome asserts, "For this reason I claim that when religious education is done by and from within a Christian community, the most descriptive term to name it is *Christian religious education*" (p. 24). In support of this supposition, any discussion in this study is also derived from the Christian faith.

Groome's (1980) descriptive definition of Christian religious education creates an awareness that the transcendent dimension does not exist in a vacuum; it is part and parcel of the innermost person (Leuba, 1969). Groome identifies Horace Bushnell, George Albert Coe, C. Ellis Nelson, and John Westerhoff, III as great Protestant theorists who promoted a socialization approach to religious education. Coe (1919) took a liberal socialist position to religious education that maximized civil engagement. Coe made several radical statements regarding the church:

> The church is necessary as a preacher of *radical* good will, which is human participation
> in divine love that, though it may be repulsed, will not be defeated. The church is
> necessary as a champion of the 'forlorn hopes' of society, the social causes that the
> 'practical' man regards as visionary. The church is necessary, finally as an educator
> of children in these ideals and practices. It is the only institution of large scope that

we can have any hope of inducing to teach democracy in this thoroughgoing fashion. Liberalism needs the church for the achievement of liberty itself. (p. 342)

Groome (1980) supports the position that "Social interaction is at the heart of Christian education not only as the process, but also as the content" (p. 118). Although socialization is critical to religious education, it must be accompanied in stages with the critique of dialectical relationships (Fowler, 1981). The development of faith in stages supports the type of gradual transformation that is possible with transformative religious education. The discussion that takes place in African-American adult religious education settings is a ripe context for intentional and transformative learning. Groome argues, "The dialectical relationship between the Christian community and its social context, and between the community and its individual members, must not be left to chance, but should be intentionally promoted" (p. 122). Adult religious education that is transformative in nature has the potential for creating such a relationship.

An assertion of this study is that adult religious education is communal with naturally occurring transcendent and transformative opportunities. Elias (1993) states, "The task of the adult religious educator is to maximize the positive attitudes and emotions of adult learners while minimizing the negative attitudes or barriers" (p. 103). Elias recognized the "need to be especially attentive to change events in the lives of learners" (p. 104). Elias' concept of adult religious education supports the transformative learning theoretical framework of this study.

Philosophies and Theories of Religious Education

Sealey (1985) identified four theories regarding the function of religious education: confessional, neo-confessional, hidden-confessional, and implicit. Confessional religious education has the teaching of Christian doctrines as its focus. "The function of RE is to extend the work of the church into the schools; to bring young people to accept the Christian religion" (p. 45). The neo-confessionists seek to develop competency in religious knowledge (p. 45). Hidden confessionists allow their students to choose their religious belief (p. 50). Finally, the implicit approach to religion involves teaching religion as part of the student's curriculum (p. 52).

Although Sealey (1985) refers to the student as a child in this discussion, it is assumed that the approaches are also used in adult religious education as well. On the other hand, Elias (1993) presents theoretical approaches to adult religious education from the perspective of adult learning philosophies: liberal, progressive, socialization-behavioristic, humanistic, and socio-political.

Philosophies of Adult Education

In a discussion of adult learning, Price (1999) identified the major focus of five commonly accepted philosophies:

1. "Liberal education emphasizes the development of rational, intellectual powers and the transmission of organized content knowledge through disciplinary study" (p. 3).
2. Progressive adult education "serves principally to facilitate learning processes by organizing, guiding and evaluating learning experiences while engaged in such experiences him or herself" (p. 4).

3. Behaviorist adult education as an "overarching purpose of education is to ensure the survival of individuals, the human species and society. . . . Educational behaviorism focuses on observable, measurable behavior and emphasizes the control of behavior through the manipulation of environmental conditions" (p. 4).

4. "Humanistic adult education sets goals for the holistic development of persons toward their fullest potential" (p. 4).

5. Radical adult education views "education as a requisite vehicle to fundamental and profound social change in economic and political spheres" (p. 4).

Of these five orientations to adult learning, the humanistic view is more closely aligned with a transformative approach to adult religious education, although not at the exclusion of viable components from the other four approaches.

▪ *Adult Learning Theories*

Learning is said to be an elusive process that is hard to define; however, there is consensus that learning is gained from experience and ultimately leads to some type of permanent change. "Learning from experience involves adults connecting what they have learned from current experiences to those in the past as well to possible future situations" (Merriam & Caffarella, 1999, pp. 246, 248-250). For the purpose of this study, adult learning theories will be discussed in relation to religious education. According to Elias (1993), adult learning theories impact adult religious education in several ways:

1. *Behaviorist Theories.* "Programmed instruction, computer-assisted instruction, personalized systems of education, skills training, and competency-based education" (p.108).

2. *Gestalt Psychology.* "Gestaltists contend that learning comes about through the development of understanding, insight, and problem solving abilities" (p. 108).

3. *Cognitive Theories.* "Significant changes in thinking abilities, capacities, and processes occur as a function of age, experience, and intellectual sophistication" (p. 109).

4. *Psychodynamic Theory.* "The primary processes described in learning include identification with others, internalization of the values of others, resolution of internal conflict of a biological and psychosocial nature, and the learning of defense and coping mechanisms that enable persons to handle difficult emotional situations (Vaillant, 1977)" (p. 110).

5. *Social Learning Theory.* "These psychodynamically oriented learning theorists utilize such constructs as identification with others, internalization of values and behaviors, learning of dependency-independency, and learning of aggression in order to explain how learning takes place throughout life" (p. 111).

6. *Humanistic Learning Theory.* Five basic assumptions are espoused in this theory; however, "The emphasis on freedom, discovery, dialogue, and changing of perceptions is most attractive" (pp. 112-113).

7. *Freire's Theory of Conscientization.* "Knowing and learning takes place in ongoing cycles of action, reflection, critical action. The learning process is primarily one of dialogue" (p. 113).

As can be noted from the statements provided from each of these theoretical perspectives, elements of each theory seem to resonate with various components of the transformation theory, with the humanistic and conscientization theories bearing the closest similarities. Knowles (1980), Freire (1970, 1973), and Tough (1979) are a few of the prominent adult educators whose theoretical outlooks support the transformative orientation of adult religious education as put forth in this and other studies (as cited in Elias, 1993). Perhaps theories of learning, adult education, and adult religious education should be viewed tangentially, with religion as a social context that influences how life events are perceived and experienced. Amstutz (1999) offers four major dominant models for adult learning theory: behaviorist, humanist, cognitivist, and liberatory (p. 19). She offers the following critique:

> All four views of adult learning often exclude the types of learning that best suit some women, people of color, and people from the working class or those who are unemployed. Other factors that affect adult learning can and should be developed and fostered to promote a more equitable society... current adult learning theory may not lead to effective learning for many adults, especially ethnic or racial minorities and women. (pp. 19-20)

Amstutz's theoretical perspective is one of emancipatory learning, where knowledge is contextual and liberating. In concert with Amstutz's viewpoint, Thompson (2000) correlated emancipatory learning with critical thinking and transformation—which are two concepts related to this study. In her discussion of emancipatory learning, Thompson writes:

> The radical tradition in adult learning is concerned with how learning, knowledge and education can be used to assist individuals and groups to overcome educational disadvantage, combat social exclusion and discrimination, and challenge economic and political inequalities—with a view to securing their own emancipation and promoting progressive social change. (Abstract)

Thus, another premise of the current study is that adult religious education is emancipatory, possessing both contextual and liberating qualities. Elias (1993) provides a comprehensive overview of the relationship between religion and the following theories of adult education: liberal, progressive, socialization-behavioristic, humanistic, socio-political (pp. 151-176; also see Sealey, 1985). Amstutz finds relevance for religious education in each of the theoretical approaches, which support the notion of "no line of demarcation" as put forth by Dewey (1933) regarding his discourse on *thinking* (p. 9).

▓ Religion, Spirituality, and Health

According to Fontana (2003), "Religion has been one of the major formative influences upon human thought and behavior throughout the centuries" (p. 1). Fontana examined positive and negative effects of religion in his discussion on the psychology of religion, but concluded "Religion is a powerful and moral imperative" (p. 42). A review of literature in various fields is replete with studies that validate a positive relationship between religious/spiritual coping and health.

A study by Tisdale (2001) supports the importance of spirituality as "one of the ways people construct knowledge and meaning" (p. 233). Thus, the consensus for a positive effect of religion and spirituality on health is high in the areas of psychology (Maton, 2001; Mattis, 2002), religion (Collins,

1990; Siegel & Schrimshaw, 2002), and health (Culliford, 2002; Flannelly, Flannelly, & Weaver, 2002; Henderson, Gore, Davis, & Condon, 2003). These studies signify only a minuscule representation of the research conducted in the areas of psychology, religion, and health. However, findings indicate tremendous support for the current researcher's belief that involvement in corporate and private religious/spiritual activities is pivotal to the wellbeing of African-American women. Thus, an overall sense of health and well-being is the expected outcome of effective adult religious education or religious involvement (Ellison, 1990; Ellison, Boardman, Williams, & Jackson, 2001; Ellison & Gay, 1990; George, Ellison, & Larson, 2002). According to Musgrave et al. (2002), "Taken together or separately, religiosity and spirituality provide a framework for making sense of the world and coping with life." (p. 557).

▓ *Religious Participation and Transformative Learning*

Musgrave et al. (2002) and Wiley et al. (2002) support the premise that participation in religious activities helps African-American women cope with the challenges of life. According to Musgrave et al., "Prayer, the Bible, and the church community are the resources religious Black women use to meet daily needs" (p. 558). Wiley et al. (2002) found that "prayer was the most common coping mechanism, and as troubles became more serious, people responded that prayer is even more helpful" (p. 265).

In the current researcher's personal pastoral experiences, she had found that in most instances, parishioners request prayer above anything else. Prayer is especially requested for hospitalized and homebound patients. According to Mattis (2002), prayer is the spiritual discipline most used by African-American women as a coping resource (p. 309). Research supports the premise that perspective transformation is within itself a means of coping because of its reflective nature, which also relates to the nature of prayer. Prayer as a spiritual discipline can motivate one to change based on personal beliefs about the power of prayer.

Belief systems. According to Mezirow (2000), "Formulating more dependable beliefs about our experience, assessing their contexts, seeking informed agreement on their meaning and justification and making decisions on the resulting insights are central to the adult learning process" (p. 4). Thus, one's belief system is foundational to how one learns and makes sense of life experiences, which involves a particular function of reflection. Thus, transformative learning demands a reassessment of the presuppositions on which our beliefs are based. Furthermore, it may involve correcting distorted assumptions from prior learning (Mezirow 1990, p. 18).

Culture. The communal and cultural contexts of the African-American church may provide the interactive characteristics necessary for transformative learning in adults. Perhaps these are a few of the essential components of transformative learning that will set the stage for the kind of meaning-making that leads to change, offering a canopy from which to view adult religious education experiences in the African-American church (Walsh, 1999).

Experience. My personal experiences as an ordained (African-American female) Protestant minister, adult educator, and religious educator lead me to believe that the communal and cultural contexts of adult religious education in the African-American church serve as a catalyst for ushering in the integration of factors necessary for critical reflection and meaning-making in transformative learning. The integration of "our urgent need to understand and order the meaning of our experience . . . to avoid the threat of chaos" (Mezirow, 2000, p. 3) places critical reflection and meaning-making at the helm of coping in general and religious coping in particular. After all, religion/spirituality's major function does seem to be one of ordering one's life.

Critical reflection. Since the very nature of adult religious education could lend itself to the process that addresses contextual and cultural aspects of transformative learning, the role of discernment and critical reflection and their relationship to ordering one's life are significant to this study. The researcher proposes that adult religious education is a source from which the integration of critical reflection and mean making are drawn to effect coping abilities in African-American women as they play out their roles in various relationships.

According to Schaller (1996), "A different view of transformation, one that more accurately reflects women's experience, is needed. Women's growth as persons is tied more to making connections than to severing relationships, even with themselves" (section on Transformation and Mentoring, para. 2). Perhaps the church is the one place where African-American women might be able to safely engage this process of meaning-making that is gained through and nourished by her participation in adult religious education.

Basically, the teaching of Christian principles in predominantly African-American churches provides a homogeneous environment where participants are more likely to trust and share, qualities that are essential for critical reflection and meaning-making (Ellison, 1990; Krause, Ellison, & Marcum, 2002). Trust is particularly important since women are likely to disclose feelings about their common journey—a journey in which they are subject to similar life experiences or "struggles" related to class, ethnicity, gender, and cultural differences. Perhaps the "struggles" themselves are enough to trigger the kind of critical reflection needed for perspective transformation.

Mezirow (1990) makes the assertion that, "to make meaning means to make sense of an experience; we make an interpretation of it" (p. 1). This process of interpreting experience through the learning that comes from reflection is vital to the emancipatory and transformative nature of adult religious education. According to Mezirow, "Reflection enables us to correct distortions in our beliefs and errors in problem solving. Critical reflection involves a critique of the presuppositions on which our beliefs have been built" (p. 1). Since adult religious practices greatly inform the Christian's basic belief system, it is essential that adult educators and other educators of adult learners explore more critically the relationships that exist between adult religious education and other forms of adult learning.

▨ Summary

This researcher questions the relationship between coping and religious practices. She will use this study to explore how one's religious and spiritual experiences affect change in meaning perspectives and lifestyle, as well as change in coping resources following disruptive life crises. Tisdale (2000) found that "adult learners bring their whole selves, including their spirituality, with them when they enter the learning environment" (p. 332). Thus, this study engages the transformative learning process from a spiritual dimension—adult religious education—and supports Mezirow's (1991) view that transformative learning demands a critical evaluation of one's life scripts if change is to occur.

The literature review discussed transformation theory and transformative learning as essential to the human situation (Dworkin, 1959), which indicates that the adult learner grows and changes every day—as supported by Taylor's 1997 empirical studies that critiqued Mezirow's transformative learning theory.

Four major topics were explored as a result of this review. First, transformation theory was discussed as the theoretical framework for this current study. Definitions of transformative learning and perspective transformation were explained, and stages of perspective transformation were applied to the life of Saint Paul of the New Testament. Issues regarding meaning-making, discernment of the transcendent, and frame of reference and the adult learner were acknowledged. Second, a brief review of stress and coping assessment and strategies was addressed, with prayer identified as the key coping resource. Examples of how prayer was used in the life of Harriet Tubman and Hagar of the Old Testament were presented along with ways in which African-American women make meaning through commitments and relationships. Third, philosophies and theories of religious education and adult education were discussed within the context of adult learning. Fourth, the concepts of belief systems, culture, experience, and reflection were examined from the perspective of religious/spirituality, and health. Studies revealed a positive relationship between religious-based coping and well-being.

The roles of religious participation and transformation in adult learning reflect positive relationships. Participation in religious activities was found to aid coping abilities in African-American women; perspective transformation was found to have coping qualities. In conclusion, the review of the literature suggests that African-American women often turn to religious coping as a means of managing stress, and that certain religious experiences can lead to a perspective transformation.

CHAPTER III
METHODOLOGY

▨ Sampling

A convenience sampling was utilized for this study. Participants consisted of 126 African-American women volunteers between 21 and 83 years of age. The process for selecting churches and volunteers consisted of placing the church names (written on individually folded slips of paper of uniform size) of approximately fifty local African-American Protestant churches in southeast Mississippi (Hattiesburg-Pine Belt area) in a container and drawing out ten churches.

Ten churches were selected and contacted via telephone to confirm their willingness to participate. One church elected not to participate in the study. Another church's name was pulled from the container and contacted. Once all ten churches committed verbally to participating, a letter requiring the pastor's signature on the agency consent form was mailed via the United States Post Office; other follow-up letters of thanks, confirmation, instruction, and information were also mailed (Bishop, 2006, Appendix A).

Consenting participants were solicited from the churches that were selected (Bishop, 2006, Appendix B). With the researcher present, the pastor or designated church representative of each church asked women 21 years old or older who were interested in taking the survey to sign up with the church secretary or women ministry leader. The pastor or designated church representative highlighted the purpose of the study from the information he or she had already received in the package provided by the researcher. Upon telephone confirmation of the established date and location for the study, the researcher administered the survey to those women volunteers who expressed interest.

The researcher was an ordained female African-American Baptist minister and has participated during the last 36 months in various religious experiences (i.e., worship, Bible study, mission, revivals, and conducting retreats) at selected churches because of her own pastoral duties and spiritual formation ministry to women. Tisdale (2000) emphasized the importance of knowing one's own "positionality" (race, gender, class, etc.) in conducting research as she discussed the theoretical framework of her own study. She concluded,

> Thus, my own positionality as a White, middle-class woman who grew up Catholic
> and has tried to negotiate a more relevant **adult** spirituality in addition to the fact
> that I teach classes specifically about race, class, and gender issues were factors that
> affected the data collection and analysis processes. (p. 315)

Although the actual data collection for the pilot study and larger study were collected over a six month period of time (from January 2006 to June 2006), because of the researcher's positionality she had already been exposed to the various religious activities of African-American churches in southeast Mississippi. Therefore, she was not a *stranger* to most women who consented to participation in this study—though they may not have known her personally, they had seen her around and were generally familiar with her. It was important that the women and their pastors have some level of trust and confidence in her. The researcher's positionality helped establish this needed assurance, especially given the delicate nature of this study.

▩ Procedures and Research Design

An explanatory mixed method research design was used in this study. The major emphasis for the study was on quantitative data collection, followed by a qualitative component in the form of a follow-up interview (Creswell, 2005). According to Creswell, "The combination of both forms of data provides a better understanding of a research problem than one type of data alone" (p. 53). Permissions to reprint materials are found in the original dissertation (Bishop, 2006, Appendix C). The study was conducted in 3 phases: pilot study, survey, and interview.

▩ *Phase I*

Pilot study. A pilot study using 12 participants was conducted in an effort to clarify the use of language and examine the validity of questions on the survey. According to Glesne and Peshkin (1992), "Less obvious than learning about your research questions and getting a general sense of your research setting is the need to learn how to be present in that setting" (p. 31). Ultimately, the results of the pilot study were used to modify measures and processes as necessary prior to **proceeding with the larger study.**

▩ *Phase II*

Survey. Most of the data collected for this research were quantitative and were collected in the second phase of the study. Data were collected using a four-part survey that consisted of the instruments described in the "Assessment Measures" section of this study. Each instrument was pilot tested for reliability with the selected sample. The Religious Participation Assessment scores on 12 surveys were examined over time (initial pilot and a re-test of pilot) to establish reliability since it was a newly developed instrument.

▩ *Phase III*

Interview. Five semi-structured private interview, which consisted of four open-ended questions and other probes, were conducted with participants who reflected extreme high scores or low scores (or otherwise interesting/pertinent feedback). Interviews were conducted in private follow-up sessions with the five participants who consented to the follow-up. The interviews served to prompt further discussion of results from the four-part survey. They also allowed participant and researcher alike to clarify any other relevant issues related to the study.

▓ Instruments

Four instruments were combined into a survey booklet and administered as one battery. Individual instruments contained their own set of instructions. Upon completion of the battery, each instrument was hand scored separately.

▓ *Religious Participation Assessment (RPA)*

The RPA, which was designed by the researcher, was used to collect demographic data and information on religious participation (Bishop, 2006, Appendix D). Questions on the RPA were chosen based on typical demographical information collected on other instruments. The more specific questions were included based on the researcher's experience in the field of religion and Christian education. The demographic portion of the questionnaire (questions 1 through 9 and 11 through 14) assessed age, social economic status, and level of education.

Question 10 served as a *religious participation* scale, requiring participants to assess their personal religious/spiritual involvement on two levels: Social/Corporate (church worship, Sunday school, church Bible study, church prayer meeting) and Private/Personal (personal prayer, personal Bible reading, personal witnessing, and spiritual retreat). These items were responded to using a five-point scale (4: 0 = never, 1 = few times a year, 2 = few times a month, 3 = weekly, and 4 = more than weekly). The ratings represent points assigned to that item (e.g., a participant attending worship services weekly would receive 3 points). The total number of points on both scales represented a participation score. Scale scores (Social/Corporate and the Private/Personal) allowed the researcher to further explore the relationship between scale items and the CRI and WORCS scores.

Question 15 contained a *stressful events* chart that was used to compare type of stressful events listed with type of events identified on the Social Readjustment Rating Scale (Holmes & Rahe, 1967). Items on this chart were rated on a scale of 1 to 10, with 1 representing the least stressful and 10 representing the most stressful.

Question 16 allowed participants to make additional comments. This question was qualitative in nature, allowing the participant to express herself without forced choices. Qualitative data collected here allowed participants to clarify any previous statements and to provide additional information.

The RPA was pilot tested prior to proceeding with the larger study to establish reliability information. Results from the pilot study are presented in the following section.

▓ *Social Readjustment Rating Scale (SRRS)*

The SRRS was designed by Holmes and Rahe (1967) to identify stressful life events that have occurred over the last 12 months (Bishop, 2006, Appendix E). The SRRS is a checklist measure that contained 43 yes/no responses to events that were indicative of the participant's lifestyle and that had occurred in the participant's life. The summary score served as an indicator of the level of change needed to readjust after a stressful event, which also functioned as a health risk predictor (Wethington, 2003). In the original development of the instrument, the authors defined social readjustment and instructed participants as follows:

You are asked to rate a series of life events as to their relative degrees of necessary readjustment. In scoring, *use all of your experience* in arriving at your answer. This means personal experience where it applies as well as what you have learned to be the case for others. Some persons accommodate to change more readily than others; some persons adjust with particular ease or difficulty to only certain events. Therefore, strive to give your opinion of the average degree of readjustment necessary for each event rather than the extreme. (Holmes & Rahe, 1967, p. 213)

For the purposes of this current study, the rankings reported by Holmes and Rahe (1967, p. 216) were used—with the listed mean values omitted—as a checklist for identifying stressful life events. Additionally, participants were asked to identify the number of occurrences they had experienced for each life event. The number of occurrences was multiplied by the rating assigned to that item by Holmes and Rahe in their original development of this instrument—providing a more accurate SRRS social adjustment score for that stressful event. For the purpose of this study, only the total number of occurrences was summed.

In light of the magnitude of a recent natural disaster that grossly affected local Mississippi residents who participated in this study, the researcher deemed it necessary to modify the SRRS checklist by adding a 44th item: natural disasters. The instructions for this item asked participants to rate Hurricane Katrina (August 29, 2005) on a scale of 1 to 10. The summed score of items 1 through 43 represented the number of stressful events experienced over the last year. The researcher used the pilot study to establish reliability for the SRRS for its use in this research. The Cronbach's Alpha reliability on the SRRS for this study was .73.

▦ *Coping Resources Inventory (CRI)*

The CRI is a 60-item instrument developed by Marting and Hammer (1988) for measuring coping resources in the cognitive (items 3, 6, 11, 12, 14, 18, 23, 49, and 55), social (items 4, 8, 9, 15, 25, 27, 28, 30, 35, 50, 53, 58, and 59), emotional (items 2, 7, 16, 17, 19, 24, 29, 31, 34, 37, 39, 40, 45, 47, 54, and 57), spiritual/philosophical (10, 20, 22, 32, 33, 38, 41, 44, 46, 48, and 52), and physical domains (items 1, 5, 13, 21, 26, 36, 42, 43, 51, 56, and 60) (Bishop, 2006, Appendix F).

CRI items were presented on a 4-point scale that was scored by simply summing all responses on each scale. The scales contained six reverse score items (5, 36, 49, 51, 58, and 59). Marting and Hammer reported a Cronbach's Alpha total internal consistency score of .91 for various samples using this instrument (p. 17). The Cronbach's Alpha standardized reliability on the CRI for this study was .92.

Scores on the CRI indicated the type of resources currently used by participants for stress management. According to Marting and Hammer (1988), "The CRI was constructed to facilitate an emphasis on resources rather than deficits. Identifying and acknowledging clients' resources and competencies as well as their deficits and impairments may prove useful in designing interventions and in improving self-concept" (p. 1). High and low scores on this profile were examined—with the assumption that high scores indicated more available coping resources.

■ *Ways of Religious Coping Scale (WORCS)*

The WORCS was designed by Boudreaux, Catz, Ryan, Amaral-Melendez, and Brantley (1995) to assess the use of religion in coping with stress (Bishop, 2006, Appendix G). The WORCS contained 40 likert-type items that measure Internal/Private and External/Social factors. Boudreaux et al. (1995) reported a Cronbach Alpha = .95 was for reliability: Internal/Private scale (.97) and External/Social scale (.93). The sum of items 1, 5, 12, 14, 16, 24, 28, 31, 32, 33, 34, 35, 37, and 38 comprised the Internal/Private scale. The sum of items 7, 8, 17, 20, 25, 26, 29, 30, 36, and 40 encompassed the External/Social scale.

The remaining items (2, 3, 4, 9, 10, 11, 13, 18, 21, 22, and 27) on the scale were not used to determine validity or reliability of the instrument. All items were rated on a 5-point likert scale: 0 = not at all/does not apply, 1 = used sometimes, 2 = used often, 3 = used very often, and 4 = used always. Reverse scoring was used on four items: 6, 19, 23, and 39). For standardized items, the Cronbach's Alpha reliability for this study was .92.

■ *Follow-Up Interview Questions*

How did religious activities, relationships, social services, or other organizations help you cope with stressful life events you experienced during the last 6 to 12 months? Identify the three most helpful agencies and rate each on a scale of 1 (LOW) to 10 (HIGH).Are there any important changes in how you feel, think, or act because of these stressful event that led you to change your lifestyle or religious practices? _____ No. _____ Yes. If yes, explain.

If you answered YES to question three above, which stressful event triggered this change? Will the change be permanent?

■ *Summary*

In summary, the RPA was used to collect various demographic information and to assess the level of involvement in religious/spiritual activities. Second, SRRS served to identify the type and number of major stressors experienced over the last year. Third, the CRI was used to determine the type of coping resources currently used by participants for managing stress. Fourth, the WORCS identified ways in which religion was used as a resource for coping. Finally, follow-up interviews were conducted to further probe findings derived from surveys. Results derived from surveys and interviews are presented in chapter 4 of this study.

■ Pilot Study Results

The major purpose of the pilot study was to clarify the use of language and examine the reliability of questions on the four-part survey. Secondly, the pilot was conducted to field test the RPA prior to proceeding with the larger study to establish reliability. The results of the pilot study resulted in a few minor changes in the instruments selected for use in this research.

The two questions that presented confusion were examined and necessary modifications were made (1. On Q44 of the SRRS, the rating scale was reversed to reflect 1 = lowest and 10 = highest and "place a check to the right of stressors affected by Katrina" was omitted; 2. On Q21 of the CRI, 2 kg was changed to 5 lbs). The test-retest for reliability for the RPA was .85. Means and standard deviations are listed in Table 1.

▓ Data Collection

The researcher used a mixed method approach, which included a four-part survey with qualitative elements and a semi-structured follow-up interview. With the researcher present during a church service, the pastors or a designated church representative announced the study by reading an excerpt of the stated purpose from the informational materials previously received. Women who were interested in the study were asked to contact the church and wait for a scheduled survey time. Once the survey administration date and place was established, this was announced publicly. Interested women met at the designated date and time with the researcher. Upon arriving at the site, the researcher was introduced to the group prior to proceeding with the survey. Each participant was given a copy of the Cover Letter and the Oral Presentation (Bishop, 2006, Appendices J and K, respectively).

Table 1

Means and Standard Deviations for Pilot Study Test-Retest for Reliability

	N	Minimum	Maximum	M	SD
Partici_1	12	20.00	25.00	22.92	1.62
Partici_2	12	21.00	28.00	23.50	2.28

After reading the Oral Presentation the researcher had the participants to complete the Informed Consent prior to administering the four-part questionnaire that included the RPA, SRRS, CRI, and the WORCS. Each participant completed the survey at her own speed and returned it to the researcher. Because of structural repairs and church renovations, some churches were not able to complete surveys onsite. Therefore, surveys that were taken home for completion were either picked up at a later date or mailed back to the researcher. Actual survey completion time was less than 1 hour per participant. Most participants took about 45 minutes to complete the survey.

Once collected, to ensure full confidentiality in the handling of data, participants' names were removed from the questionnaires, and numbers were assigned for identification purposes. Consent forms with identifying survey information were locked in a safe. After completion of the study the survey sheets will be shredded.

In collaboration with the 10 pastors at the 10 participating churches, the researcher scheduled appropriate days and times for data collection. Upon meeting the participants, the researcher introduced herself appropriately and continued with the study per instructions that were approved by the University of Southern Mississippi's Institutional Review Board (IRB). For convenience in scoring and participant response tracking, the four-part questionnaire was printed as one document.

The follow-up interviews took approximately 1 hour per interview. The potential interviewees were contacted regarding their interest in participating in the follow-up study. With their consent, arrangements were made for time and location in conducting the interview session using the

Interview Protocol designed by the researcher (Bishop, 2006, Appendix H). Upon establishing rapport in order to establish trust and open communication with the participant, the researcher proceeded with the interview—tape recording and taking handwritten notes as appropriate during the process (Creswell, 2005; Glesne & Peshkin, 1992). Interview results were thematically coded by the interviewer/researcher.

▓ Data Analysis

Multiple correlations and Pearson correlations were used to explore the relationship between variables identified in this study. First, current marital status combined single and widow to form the single category. Second, years of church membership were categorized into two groups: churchlow = 6 years to 16 years and churchmid = 16 years and up. Third, income level was also separated into two groups: incomelow = under $20,000 and incomemid = over $20,000. Fourth, levels of education were grouped to form four categories: (a) high = elementary, middle, and high school/GED; (b) some college = technical/vocational, and some college; (c) undergraduate = Associate and Bachelor Degrees; and (d) graduate = Master's Degree, Specialist Degree, and Doctoral Degree.

Pearson correlations that were examined consisted of (1) RPA total scores with RPA scale scores, (2) RPA totals scores with CRI total scores, (3) RPA total scores with WORCS total scores, and (4) CRI total scores with WORCS total scores.

The independent quantitative variables (RPA and SRRS scores) were used to explore their relationship with several dependent quantitative variables (CRI, WORCS, age, marital status, residence, number of people in household, income level, education level, and years of current church membership). Narratives from the interviews were thematically coded using the CDC EZ-Text coding system (Carey, Wenzel, Reilly, Sheridan, & Steinberg, 1997).

■ CHAPTER IV ■
DATA ANALYSIS

■ Introduction

Is participation in adult religious education a predictor of the type of coping resources used by African-American women? Is there a relationship between stressful life events, certain demographic variables, and the use of coping resources? These are the basic questions that were explored in this analysis of data. Initially, a descriptive analysis of data is presented. Second, correlation results exploring the relationship between religious participation and the use of coping resources were followed by a more specific correlation that examines the association between religious participation and religious coping. Third, relationships between stressful life events and several demographic variables were investigated using multiple regression analyses. Finally, a discussion of follow-up interview results and other qualitative data is discussed—with an emphasis on extreme scores and Hurricane Katrina.

■ Descriptive Analysis of Data

Participants for this study were volunteers from 10 randomly selected Protestant churches in southeast Mississippi. Participants (n = 126) completed a four-part survey that consisted of the Religious Participation Assessment (RPA), the Social Readjustment Rating Scale (SRRS), the Coping Resources Inventory (CRI), and the Ways of Religious Coping Scale (WORCS). In addition to the four-part survey, five participants also gave consent to be interviewed. The follow-up interviews were designed to further investigate qualitative responses and extreme scores. An alpha level of .05 was used for all statistical tests.

The sample consisted of 126 African-American women between the ages of 21 and 83 years (mean age = 44.17). Approximately 37% were single/widow, 44% were married, and 20% were divorced. Forty-five percent of the women earned incomes less than $20,000 and 29% earned between $20,000 and $40,000. A large majority of the women (81%) lived in houses/mobile homes and 18% lived in apartments.

Educational levels are presented in Table 2. Of the women surveyed, 66% had studied at the college level; approximately 47% of this group had earned college degrees. The majority (66%) of the women who participated in this study had been a member of their current church for less than 20 years; approximately 29% boasted of holding membership in the same church for more than 20 years. In fact, the longest standing membership in the same church was reported at 78 years.

Table 2

Frequency for Level of Education

	Frequency	Percent
Middle School	5	4.0
High School/GED	29	23.0
Technical/Vocational	3	2.4
Some College	29	23.0
Associate's Degree	16	12.7
Bachelor's Degree	26	20.6
Master's Degree	16	12.7
Specialist Degree	1	.8
Total	125	100.0

▦ Correlations for Religious Participation and Coping

The Pearson product-moment correlation coefficient (r) was used to determine the relationship between religious participation (RPA), the use of general coping (CRI), and the use of religious coping resources (WORCS). Results are presented in Table 3.

Table 3

Pearson Correlations for Religious Participation and Coping Variables

	RPA	CRI	WORCS
RPA	1		
CRI	.208*	1	
WORCS	.355**	.391**	1

Note. RPA = Religious Participation Assessment; CRI_TOTAL = Coping Resources Inventory; WORCS = Ways of Religious Coping Scale.
$n = 126$. $df = 125$.
* $p < .05$. ** $p < .01$.

First, a low correlation, but statistically significant relationship ($r = .208$, $p < .02$), was found between RPA and CRI scores. Secondly, a moderate correlation between RPA and WORCS scores was found to be statistically significant ($r = .355$, $p < .001$).

Weak, but statistically significant correlations, were found between the CRI total and the RPA Corporate/Social Scale ($r = .185$, $p < .04$) and RPA Private/Personal Scale ($r = .178$, $p < .05$). Thus, corporate religious participation accounted for approximately 3% ($r^2 = .034$) of general coping, while the practice of private spiritual disciplines accounted for approximately 5% ($r^2 = .032$) of general coping.

Third, a positive relationship between participation in adult religious education and the use of religious coping strategies was found. Statistically significant moderate associations were found between the correlational analyses of the WORCS score, the RPA Corporate/Social Scale ($r = .319$, $p < .001$) and the RPA Private/Personal Scale ($r = .301$, $p < .001$). In this assessment, Corporate religious participation accounted for approximately 10% ($r^2 = .102$) of religious coping and personal religious participation accounted for approximately 9% ($r^2 = .091$).

Lastly, the correlation between the WORCS scores and the CRI scores was found to be moderate and statistically significant ($r = .391$, $p < .001$). Religious participation accounted for approximately 15% ($r^2 = .153$) of general coping. Means and standard deviations are shown in Table 4.

Table 4
Means and Standard Deviations for RPA, RPA Scales, CRI, and WORCS

	Mean	SD	*n*
RPA	20.42	4.83	126
RPA (Corporate Scale)	10.23	2.57	126
RPA (Private Scale)	10.19	2.98	126
CRI	83.51	24.02	126
WORCS	162.06	23.56	126

Correlations Between Stressful Events and Demographics

Correlations were computed between the SRRS scores and several demographic variables. Age was found to have a statistically significant negative relationship with stressful life events on the SRRS, $r = -.245$, $r^2 = .060$, $p < .05$). The number of stressful events experienced reflected a decrease with age. Younger people tended to experience more stressful life events than did older adults. No statistically significant relationships were evidenced for the other variables; however, weak correlations were noted (Table 5).

Table 5
Correlation of SRRS with Demographic and Educational Variables

	Age	Marital	Residence	Household	Income	Education	Church
SRRS	-.245	.169	.130	.206	.179	.137	.076
	p < .05	*ns*	*ns*	*ns*	*ns*	*ns*	*ns*

Note: All correlations except age and household were multiple correlations.

Table 6 represents challenging events that were compiled from short answer responses to questions 15 and 16 on the RPA. The major concerns were health and family (19%). The second most concern was Hurricane Katrina (14%). The third highest ranking (12%) stressor was Lifestyle—which was related to property lost, extreme property damage, and the absence of moderate inconveniences such as electricity, gas, water and fuel (all associated with Hurricane Katrina). It is interesting to note that in cases where there was a death or illness in the immediate family, Hurricane Katrina was not given a rating or was given a lower rating than the family situation that caused stress. In a few cases that involved serious family illnesses, Hurricane Katrina was not mentioned at all.

Table 6
Frequency and Percentages of Challenging Events on RPA Q15 and Q16

Challenging Event	Total	Percentage
Death	35	9
Family	75	19
Finances	36	9
God	22	6
Health	76	19
Job	27	7
Katrina	55	14
Lifestyle	46	12
School	11	3
Transportation	8	2

■ *Participation in Adult Religious Education*

The level of participation in adult religious education activities is shown in Tables 7 – 14. The frequency for participation ranged from "never" to "nearly everyday." The four corporate activities are typically conducted on a weekly basis. The exception for worship would usually be the inclusion of a revival. Each activity listed for private involvement can de done on a daily basis; however, although personal retreat is usually done less frequently (quarterly, bi-annually, or annually), some women did it daily.

Table 7
Church Worship Service Participation Level

	Frequency	Percent
Never		
Few times a year	1	.8
Few times a month	9	7.1
Weekly	95	75.4
Nearly everyday	21	16.7
Total	126	100

Table 8
Church Sunday School Participation Level

	Frequency	Percent
Never	21	16.7
Few times a year	10	7.9
Few times a month	29	23.0
Weekly	66	52.4
Nearly everyday		
Total	126	100.00

Table 9
Church Bible Study Participation Level

	Frequency	Percent
Never	5	4.0
Few times a year	9	7.1
Few times a month	21	16.7
Weekly	86	68.3
Nearly everyday	5	4.0
Total	126	100.0

Table 10
Church Prayer Meeting Participation Level

	Frequency	Percent
Never	12	9.5
Few times a year	13	10.3
Few times a month	15	11.9
Weekly	77	61.1
Nearly everyday	8	6.3
Total	125	99.2

Table 11
Personal Prayer Participation Level

	Frequency	Percent
Never	4	3.2
Few times a year	4	3.2
Few times a month	3	2.4
Weekly	17	13.5
Nearly everyday	96	98.4
Total	124	98.4

Table 12
Personal Bible Reading Participation Level

	Frequency	Percent
Never	4	3.2
Few times a year	6	4.8
Few times a month	17	13.5
Weekly	26	20.6
Nearly everyday	72	57.1
Total	125	99.211

Table 13
Personal Witnessing Participation Level

	Frequency	Percent
Never	11	8.7
Few times a year	11	8.7
Few times a month	29	23.0
Weekly	39	31.0
Nearly everyday	36	28.6
Total	126	100.0

Table 14
Personal Spiritual Retreat Participation Level

	Frequency	Percent
Never	54	42.9
Few times a year	58	46.0
Few times a month	6	4.8
Weekly	4	3.2
Nearly everyday	3	2.4
Total	125	99.2

▣ Qualitative Analysis of Data

As a follow-up to the quantitative data collection, five semi-structured interviews were conducted privately with participants who volunteered during the survey to continue with the study should they be selected for a follow-up. Excerpts from each interview are provided in this section.

▣ *Participant #14*

This 74-year-old evangelist/missionary showed her devoutness by initially listing multiple religious activities in which she engages regularly. She spends most of her time serving the church in some capacity. She did not admit to using religion as a primary coping resource; however her total involvement in the work of her local church supports this claim. Prayer and meditation are the private/personal coping resources that she listed as her major coping strategies.

She identified church (#8) and FEMA (#9) and the major helping agencies she used during Hurricane Katrina. This participant named several organizations in which she held office. She described her conversion experience and her call to ministry, which she experienced following her conversion, as the single most stressful event. Although there were over 40 years between both experiences, these were the two most significant life events that motivated permanent changes in her lifestyle. (For excerpt of conversation, see Bishop, 2006, pp. 77-78).

▣ *Participant #61*

This participant was a 22-year-old recent college graduate who lives on the Gulf Coast in Mississippi. She lost everything she had in Hurricane Katrina. She confessed that the devastation from Hurricane Katrina completely changed her life. This young woman admitted that she turned back to God as a result of spiritual guidance she received from other people during Hurricane Katrina.

When asked how religious activities, relationships, social services, or other organizations helped her cope with stressful life events, she stated, "Religious activities brought me closer to God [during Katrina). Bible study helped me. I paid more attention at church. I have always been very stressful. Tools people gave me helped strengthen me." She identified and ranked the three most resourceful agencies that helped her through the storm as: boss (#10), sorority (#8), and church (#9). This respondent affirmed that Hurricane Katrina had triggered a permanent change in her. (For excerpt of conversation, see Bishop, 2006, pp. 78-79).

■ *Participant #77*

This interviewee was a 37-year-old church administrator who described her fulltime engagement in religious activities during Hurricane Katrina and the close relationship of a close friend as her major coping resources during the storm. In fact, her church served as a local distribution center for her city.

Participant #77 rated church families and people working together as her #10 helping agencies, followed by FEMA and the Red Cross as #8 or #9. Although she did not experience in major changes in lifestyle during this time, she does admit to falling short in her Bible reading – a feeling that she was not reading enough. The permanent lifestyle change that resulted from this woman's religious experienced was very similar to that of participant #14. However, although this participant's religious conversion experience and call to ministry came a year before her mother's death, she gives equal credit to the role each of these events played in inspiring a very permanent change that occurred in her life during that time – often referring to levels of faith as paramount to her strength and walk with God. (For excerpts of conversation, see Bishop, 2006, pp. 79-81).

■ *Participant #88*

This 50-year-old office manager placed the Word of God and praying at the center of her religious coping resources during the last year as she contended with devastation of Hurricane Katrina and her husband's job situation [self-employed with very little revenue]. She ranked FEMA #7, churches #8, and the Department of Human Services #8 as the top three most helpful resources agencies during the storm. When asked about important life changes that were prompted by Hurricane Katrina, she spoke about an increased awareness of her environment and changes in her relationship with God. (For excerpts of conversation, see Bishop, 2006, pp. 81-82).

■ *Participant #122*

This last young woman was a 42-year-old, unemployed, single mother with a handicapped child. She shared the story of her struggle with alcoholism prior to her religious conversion experience. As with a few of the other participants, when asked what her main coping resource was, she named turning to God's Word as her primary strategy: "The Word. Knowing that I can go to the Word and find solutions, having confidence in the Word, knowing that my situation will change. The Word is true and unchanging." She also identified the church as her primary (#10) helping agency, followed by employers (#8), and FEMA (#7). When asked if she had made any important and permanent changes during the last year, she spoke of an increase in affection toward others. (For excerpts of conversation, see Bishop, 2006, pp. 82-83).

■ *Summary*

Each of the interviewees had a religious/spiritual foundation in the Word of God, which indicated their belief in a power greater than themselves when it comes to dealing with the everyday and monumental stresses of life. Each one of them also listed church as a major helpful resource agency during Hurricane Katrina, which validates religion as a strategy for coping for them.

The other frequently mentioned factor, although not especially related to religious participation, that influenced coping was a relationship with another person—an almost overlooked and taken-for-granted coping resource inherent in religious participation. Participants spoke of relationships with pastors, Sunday school teachers, mission leaders, and church members in general. Each interviewee either alluded to or specifically mentioned people-based relationships throughout the interview process. In conclusion, qualitative data gathered during the interview process validated already established quantitative data.

■ Results of Data Analysis

A descriptive analysis of data was presented for 126 African-American women volunteers from 10 randomly selected African-American Protestant churches in southeast Mississippi. The majority of these women were married and either had some college or held a college degree, although most of them earned less than $20,000 annually. Pilot study results established reliability of each instrument: (1) RPA test-retest reliability = .85, (2) CRI standardized Cronbach's Alpha = .92, (3) WORCS standardized Cronbach's Alpha = .92, and (4) SRRS Cronbach's Alpha = .83. Third, Pearson correlation analyses indicated statistically significant, although low to moderate, associations, relationships between RPA and CRI and RPA and WORCS, respectively. Fourth, correlations computed between SRRS, demographic, and coping variables yielded only one notable relationship (age). Stressful life events were found to decrease as age increased. Finally, all interviewees were well-grounded in Word of God, used prayer regularly, and relied on the church and people as a primary helping resource during Hurricane Katrina and other stressful events.

◼ CHAPTER V ◼
DISCUSSION

◼ Introduction

The purpose, procedures, and findings from the research are presented in this chapter. A discussion and recommendations conclude the study. As indicated in chapter 1 of this study, a broader understanding of the associated assumptions of the transformative learning theory would contribute to the effectiveness of how adult religious education programs are developed and implemented in various adult learning contexts, with a focus on the African-American Christian community in the south. Two key research questions were addressed in this study.

First, how does the level of participation in adult religious education (church membership, church worship, church Sunday school, church Bible study, church prayer meeting, personal prayer, personal Bible reading, personal witnessing, personal spiritual retreat) relate to African-American women's coping resources (CRI score and WORCS score)? Secondly, is there a relationship between the experience of stressful life events, demographic variables (age, marital status, residence, number in household, income level, education level, and church membership), and coping resources? Optimally, this study will be used as a catalyst for building a broader knowledge base for designing viable adult religious education options that will positively and effectively impact spiritual, mental, and physical health (Tisdale, 2000). Vogel (2000) captured the essence of this proposition:

> Our spiritual lives reflect the dreams, fears, and commitments out of which we live, work, play, and pray. When we claim our spiritual selves and take responsibility for understanding and nurturing the spiritual dimension of our being, we learn to teach with a deeper sense of who we are, and to embody integrity in powerful, vulnerable ways. (p. 18)

◼ Procedures

To ensure the most valid collection of data, a mixed method research design (Creswell, 2005) was used to conduct this study during the spring of 2006. With prior approval from the University of Southern Mississippi Institution Review Board (Appendix L) and appropriate authors (Boudreaux & Catz, 1995; Holmes & Rahe, 1967; and Marting & Hammer, 1988), African-American adult women volunteers were administered a pilot study, a four-part survey, and a follow-up interview. The study was conducted in three phases: pilot study, survey, and interview. To maintain complete confidentiality of participants in this study, permissions received from the 10 participating churches were not published.

Visitations were made to the 10 participating churches periodically for two years leading up to this study. This was done so the women would be minimally familiar with the researcher prior to data collection. Given the nature of the African-American culture and the sensitivity of the topic, the researcher deemed this extra step necessary for establishing and maintaining rapport. All 126 participants voluntarily completed the RPA, SRRS, CRI, and WORCS assessment measures (Bishop, 2006, Appendices D – F). All data were hand-entered into the SPSS for quantitative data analysis using Pearson correlations and multiple regression analyses and EX-Text for qualitative data analysis for thematic coding, a process of systematically assigning labels to words and phrases for the purpose of grouping/scoring (Carey, Wenzel, Reilly, Sheridan, & Steinberg, 1997).

▦ Findings and Discussion

Eight participation factors were used in this study to examine the relationship between religious participation and coping: (a) church worship, (b) church Sunday school, (c) church Bible study, (d) church prayer meeting, (e) personal prayer, (f) personal Bible reading, (g) personal witnessing, and (h) spiritual retreat. The highest levels of participation by the women were personal prayer and personal Bible reading.

A majority of the women engaged in personal prayer (76%) and personal Bible reading (57%) more than weekly—some reported praying and reading more than once a day. This level of participation was matched only by a 75% weekly attendance rate at Sunday worship services, although weekly attendance at church Bible study and prayer meeting were 68% and 61%, respectively. The weakest levels of weekly participation in adult religious education activities were in the areas of church Sunday school (52%) and personal witnessing (31%). Finally, spiritual retreat—which is typically done on an annual basis, received an attendance rating of 46%.

Correlation coefficients computed on these factors and religious coping measures (CRI and WORCS), though positive and statistically significant, were not high. Further clarification of the reason for this low to moderate correlation would require further study. However, based on one of the findings of this study, which is not assumed to be the only factor that contributes to coping, church-going African-American women were found to consistently rely on religion as a coping strategy. This finding may also lead one to believe that participation in adult religious activities is definitely connected to the way certain adult African-American women maintain the balance among mind, body, and soul.

▦ *Motivations for Learning*

Adult religious educators can use these results to evaluate program effectiveness for women in each target area, especially those areas that reported low participation. An exploratory study with a strong qualitative component that applies Houle's (1961) motives for adults' learning would provide a starting point for increasing involvement in areas that show low participation. Houle made it clear that these motives are not mutually exclusive. There is overlap. One learning activity could satisfy all three motivations for participation in adult learning.

A class in English composition may appeal to an activity-oriented person because it offers him [her] credit, to a goal-oriented person because he [she] needs to know how to express himself [herself] to get ahead on his [her] job, and to a learning-oriented person because he [she] is concerned with making himself [herself] more skilled in one of the liberal arts, not for its value in reaching other ends but because it is good in and of itself. (p. 30)

Consequently, the parishioners who attend Sunday morning worship may all be motivated for different reasons. Yet, they are all in attendance at the same service. The same could hold true for participants of Sunday school, prayer meeting or Bible study. Regarding the personal religious/spiritual practices, this proposition could also be valid. Although the activities could very well remain the same for all persons, their reason for participating will vary depending on what motivates them to learn. Houle's (1961) depiction of the adult learners' model for motivation to learn resembles concentric circles. Although there is a common center, each circle overlaps the other at some point. For the adult learner, *presence* is the common element. They are all there—present.

According to Houle (1961), adults differ in their conception of why adults participate in continuing education:

The first, or as they will be called, the *goal-oriented*, are those who use education as a means of accomplishing fairly clear-cut objectives. The second, the *activity-oriented*, are those who take part because they find in the circumstances of the learning a meaning which has no necessary connection, and often no connection at all, with the content or the announced purposes of activity. The third, the *learning-oriented*, seek knowledge for its own sake. (pp. 15-16)

A greater understanding of why participants engage in one activity more frequently than another would assist purveyors of adult learning in the religious context in creating and implementing more intentional educational programs.

Activity-oriented. An activity-oriented learner would be more prone to attend worship services regularly. Worship service offers an escape from the mundane and a time for fellowship. Houle (1961) viewed the church as "an open and socially accepted place for meeting people and making friends" (p. 19). The nurturing of friendships through active fellowship was a common element found in all 10 participating churches. People could be observed visiting together before, during, and after worship service. Also, interviewees in this study spoke of the relationships, friendships, and fellowship they enjoyed within their church families.

Activity-oriented participants will be there for the sake of being there. They do not really care what the event is—so long as it gets them out of the house and into the crowd. This group will be certain to be aware of all the happenings at church or in the community because it gives them somewhere to go just to get away; it may simply provide a change of environment for the lonely. Education program planners who conduct assessments prior to program development would benefit from knowing the type of learners they are planning for.

Goal-oriented. The goal-oriented learner, on the other hand, might find Bible study to be more appealing. Bible study classes are typically structured to explore a topic of interest or to address a specific issue. Goal-oriented learners are purpose-driven. "The purpose is always what initiates the educational effort, and the means are selected on the basis of whether or not they will achieve that purpose" (Houle, 1961, p. 18). In all of the participating churches, the pastors taught the Bible study. In one of the participating churches, the pastor conducted an unusually interesting and focused Bible study that kept participants coming back week after week until the series was completed. (The researcher attended this particular Bible study series.) This creative pastor had just as many participants in Bible study as he had in church at worship services on Sundays. During several of visits to this congregation, the researcher noticed that the pastor always "talked up" the Bible study. The church systematically mailed out personal invitations inviting visitors to participate in the upcoming Bible study series.

Hence, pastors' active involvement could be one reason for higher participation in worship, prayer meeting, and Bible study. Sunday school in each of the churches surveyed was taught by laypersons—who often do not have theological training or who have limited theological training. (Research is needed to further explore this issue). He constantly promoted interest in the upcoming Bible study, which was always taught as a series and not as a single lesson. (Congressional studies on each of the churches surveyed in this study are recommended for further examination of the issues addressed here.)

Learning-oriented. The learning-oriented adult learner enjoys learning for the pure sake of learning. According to Houle (1961), "Each particular educational experience of the learning-oriented is an activity with a goal, but the continuity and range of such experiences make the total pattern of participation far more than the sum of its parts" (p. 14). Houle suggests a "preoccupation with learning" (p. 38) for this type learner that creates a *flow* in learning activities. Learning-oriented adults possess a strong "desire to know" (p. 25) that drives them to become lifelong learners. This type learner is likely to participate in every available activity for the opportunity to gain new knowledge. The probability is high that the learning-oriented adult would attend Worship service, Sunday school, prayer meeting, and Bible study weekly (along with any other meetings or special programs). They do not want to miss anything. These are the *regulars*—the ones that can be seen every time the church doors open. Regardless to why adults participate in religious education, it can be assumed that at some point they will come to question previously held values and belief systems. After all, that is one function of religion.

Implications for Transformative Learning

The researcher believes the dynamic transcendence of religious involvement to be conducive to perspective transformation. The experiences common to worship and other activities in the participating African-American churches were lively and thought provoking. Parishioners were not passive onlookers. They were actively engaged in various elements of worship and learning—the type of engagement that promotes critical reflection (as evidenced by the questions and discussions that followed). Mezirow (1991) views transformative learning as a by-product of critical analysis that involves a re-assessment of one's previously held beliefs. This assessment of transformative learning supports this researcher's belief that experiences in adult religious education create an atmosphere that could lead to critically analyzing one's typical way of thinking or behaving. The minister is often present at most important events: marriage, birth, dedication, baptism, celebrations, sickness, imprisonment, and death.

Many facets of American society acknowledge that there is a greater power that helps regulate life as we know it. After all, for some, the religious context is usually reserved as a sacred place—a type of secret closet where no one else can enter without invitation to one's space, thoughts, reflections, or other conscious/unconscious bidding.

As a minister and educator, the researcher often served as an adult religious educator, with development of the spiritual life as a principal objective. In the capacity of minister as educator, it was often necessary for her to involve many different aspects of life in the effort to establish a point or present a truth. The researcher's teaching experience in the area of adult religious education is not limited to "spiritual experiences." It has often been necessary for her to include examples or cases from the social, political, and school environments. There have also been times when representatives from various community agencies were invited to speak on religious programs that involved health, finances, politics, and other topics common to a culture.

Therefore, the holistic nature of adult learning in various religious education settings can serve as a catalyst for facilitating change—change as a result of critically re-assessing one's values and beliefs. The values and beliefs of adult learners in spiritual settings is potentially challenged when a Bible concept or lesson conflicts with the way the learner thinks, believes, or behaves. Perhaps it is this very introspection that makes religious coping a primary strategy of choice for African-American women.

According to Isaac, Guy, and Valentine (2001), "Religious coping methods include seeking spiritual support, collaborative religious coping, and spiritual connection" (p. 34). Women who were interviewed in this study shared conversion stories that placed their experiences within the context of transformative learning. Transformative learning leads to a change in "meaning perspective." According to Mezirow (1978), "A meaning perspective refers to the structure of cultural assumptions within which new experience is assimilated to—and transformed by—one's past experience" (p. 101). The main context for the conversion experiences of women interviewed in this study was the African-American church. The interviewees talked of life changing experiences. They spoke of their lives not being the same as a result of their new faith journey and the devastation from Hurricane Katrina.

> Teaching and learning that are holistic must be open to and reckon with the spiritual lives of both adult educators and learners; educators must design processes that invite the involvement of whole persons while honoring the experience of each person in ways that leave room for diversity and mystery. (Vogel, 2000, p. 17).

Vogel seems to be calling for adult educators to be fully engaged in the teaching process. In a sense, the researcher perceives this holist engagement as a call to adventuresome adult learning. The diversity and mystery of the African-American churches that participated in this survey provided ripe settings for adventuresome learning. There was as much diversity in the pastors' leadership style in these churches as there was in the overall composition of the churches themselves. Much diversity was found in ethnic backgrounds, occupations, and style of worship from congregation to congregation.

Are people more different than they are alike or more alike than they are different? The Hurricane Katrina disaster of 2005 created a sort of level playing field that tested many people on this issue of sameness and difference. The rich and poor alike were standing in long lines waiting on scarce resources; it was a time of having money and not being able to buy.

One of the interviewees for this study said it best: "People help people the best" (participant #77). While coding qualitative data, the one helping agency that each interviewee mentioned was the church. The church and the families (i.e., relationships) that serve the church proved to be a much greater force to reckon with than the giant bureaucrats. A lot of little people can get a lot of little stuff done that really matters. So it is with matters of the mind and spirit, the steadfast participation in weekly adult religious education activities can serve in the development of lasting bonds between women who position themselves for the creation of new relationships.

Relationships. Pargament (1997) saw the role of relationships as crucial to the meaning-making process. In fact, relationships are so crucial that God said that it was not good for man to be alone and he made woman: "It is not good for the man to be alone. I will make a helper suitable for him" (Genesis 2:18, NIV). People need people. When participants responded to the short answer questions in this study, they placed family (usually associated with health issues) and their own health as first priority (both at 19%). This clearly speaks to the fact that life cannot exist within a vacuum. People do need people. Although Hurricane Katrina remains fresh in the hearts and minds of some, fellowship with people in the church, family, and other settings clearly take first place in the heart of people.

According to Isaac, Guy, and Valentine (2001), "Comfort arose from the opportunity to engage in learning with other Christians and with people who had similar interests and ethnic/racial backgrounds" (p. 28). This may be one of the reasons why many churches across America remain segregated in the 21st century. Nevertheless, regardless of the congregation's diversity of similarities, when the mystery of the transcendent encounters people in worship, the door is left open for a transformative learning experience—however unconscious it may be. The transformative learning experience is not necessarily the result of a single incident; rather, it is the culmination of the total worship or educational experience. Conversations with some of the interviewees in this study affirmed a need for people to learn from each other on religious matters. Participant #61 confessed that religious activities brought her closer to God and that Bible study also helped her. Thus, a closer examination of transformative learning in the religious context is needed. Adult religious education is inundated with programs that attract people to the church. Why? Is adult religious education a type of transformative learning that leads to perspective transformation over time?

Religious experiences. Findings from this study suggest that adult religious education is a type of transformative learning that leads to perspective transformation. Religious conversion experiences shared by interviewees in this study seemed to have acted as catalysts for change (disorienting dilemmas) in their lives. Nonetheless, the consistent participation in adult religious education over the years also suggests a type of ongoing transformation (i.e., spiritual formation) that cannot be associated with any specific events; rather, the various experiences over the years would appear to have a cumulative effect on behavior, attitudes, and beliefs.

Therefore, the need for a micro-orientation to transformative learning, as espoused by Mezirow (2000), demands an examination of the role of several distinct, but similar, elements deemed imperative to transformative learning in the religious context: meaning-making, reflection, discernment, intuition, and transcendence. To gain a more inclusive view of transformative learning, these motifs must be explored within the context of various collective and individual religious/spiritual experiences—realizing the importance of experience in the lives of adult learners. The concept of *andragogy* is based on several assumptions that distinguish the adult learner from the child learner. One assumption is that "the adult accumulates a growing reservoir of experience, which is a rich resource for learning" (Knowles, 1980, p. 43). In the case of adult religious education, experience is often a combined cyclical interaction of the sacred with the secular. Parishioners bring their personal experiences from home and community into the church—experiences that are magnified and sometimes clarified under the influences of the church milieu. It is this magnification and clarification that spur meaning-making.

Meaning-making. Meaning-making, reflection, discernment, intuition, and transcendence can each be defined independently; although they are separate but related terms, the researcher considers them essential to transformative learning in the religious context. The effort to make sense of ones experiences involves the application of each of these terms. "To make meaning means to make sense of an experience; we make an interpretation of it. When we subsequently use this interpretation to guide decision making or action, then making meaning becomes learning" (Mezirow, 1990, p. 1). When viewed from the standpoint of adult religious education as transformative learning, these terms have integrative value. Each term places a demand on the adult learner to critically evaluate, reconstruct, discard, or incorporate some belief or behavior.

Reflection. Reflection requires a critical looking back on turning from some thought, belief, or action. Discernment creates a need for comprehending uncertain situations involving ambiguous thoughts or actions. Intuition involves acquiring knowledge without evidence. Transcendence indicates some internal and mysterious knowledge of God. The process of meaning-making places a demand on the learner to construct relative meaning out of chaos by integrating qualities from each of the terms discussed, especially when learning is located in a sacred communal setting.

The researcher understands a sacred communal setting to be a place where one experiences (or is engulfed by) the presence of God in a way that transcends natural human understanding. Participant #77 described such an atmosphere when she discussed her spiritual experiences during our interview. Her nonverbal expression and intonation added meaning to the conversation that she could not vocalize. She tried without success to articulate what it was like to speak in tongues and be filled with the Holy Spirit. She kept motioning with her hands and face and grasping for words to communicate the thoughts that were beyond her comprehension, thoughts that would not form no matter how she reflected back on the experience. Her effort to make sense or meaning of the conversion experience left her with only her intuition. She knew what she knew although she did not know how she knew it. Nothing in the repertoire of her experience had prepared her for this disorienting dilemma that was evoked by her religious experience—an experience that happened within the adult religious education context of worship. The transcendent influence at operation in this experience may not have been at the conscious level for this participant.

This participant (#77) confessed that a permanent change had taken place in her life because of her conversion experience, indicating a perspective transformation. This young woman had—by virtue of the change described—challenged her previously held assumptions about what it meant to be a Christian. Her efforts to make meaning of her new experience worked as a catalyst for change that inevitably involved some of the key concepts discussed in this study: meaning-making, reflection, discernment, intuition, and transcendence.

Upon evaluation of the means of religious participation, some participants wrote in the word *meditation*. Meditation can be seen as a form of reflection that involves transcendence in that the attainment of understanding gained through meditation cannot be achieved without employing reflection. Thus, meditation in this study serves as a religious resource that can serve as a strategy for coping with stress. "Reflection enables us to correct distortions in our beliefs and errors in problem solving" (Mezirow, 1990, p. 1). The corrective quality of critical reflection may be the reason meditation was listed as a coping strategy. If so, then it would be beneficial for religious educators, therapists, and healthcare agencies to actively incorporate the use of meditation and other related spiritual disciplines in a holistic approach to women's wellness. Houle (1961) perceived participation in church to be "a kind of preventive psychiatric role" (p. 19). In other words, participation in church plays a therapeutic role in the lives of parishioners. Those women interviewed during the follow-up made references to the calming effect of spiritual retreats and how they are able to think clearer after the retreats. A few participants reported engaging in daily retreat time for communion with God.

Participant #14 specifically mentioned the use of spiritual retreat and meditation as a personal coping strategy. She talked of not being able to understand what was happening on the inside of her (a transcendent experience that exceeded her normal ability to comprehend). This participant (as well as other interviewees) clearly used meditation to help make sense of the internal changes she was experiencing. It is difficult for me to comprehend the use of meditation without the simultaneous use of reflection.

> Reflection would include making inferences, generalizations, analogies, discriminations, and evaluations, as well as feeling, remembering, and solving problems. It also seems to refer to using beliefs to make an interpretation, to analyze, perform, discuss, or judge—however unaware one may be of doing so. (Mezirow (1990, p. 5).

This exposition on the meaning of reflection by Mezirow points to two closely related terms that incorporate similar qualities: discernment and intuition.

Discernment. Discernment was defined in chapter 1 of this study as "the quality of being able to grasp and comprehend what is obscure" (Mish et al., 1999, p. 330). The ambiguity involved in reflection mirrors the obscurity of discernment and intuition. The meaning of each concept— reflection, discernment, and intuition—supports the notion that adult religious education has transcendent properties essential to a transformative learning experience.

Intuition. Mish et al. (1999) defined intuition as "an act of contemplating" and as "the power or faculty of attaining to direct knowledge or cognition without evident rational thought and inference" (p. 615). Intuition is commonly referred to as a sixth sense. There is a sense of knowing that is not based on anything concrete. You just know that you know—not understanding how you know. There is an element of transcendence present with intuition. Adult learners' life experiences may be a contributing factor to what they call intuition. Perhaps stored memories that are unconscious to the learner play an active role in this sense of *knowing without knowing*. It is feasible to think that the accumulation of years of life experiences can be active in the subconscious mind, waiting on the opportune moment to manifest itself in the form of new (although unknown) knowledge. The discussion of transcendence that follows is closely related to this topic.

Transcendence. According to Coyle (2002), transcendence is defined as: (a) *intrapersonal*, a type of inner knowledge of God; and (b) *transpersonal*, a connectedness with God based on *meaning* and *purpose* with other people (p. 590). In this study, approximately 46% of all participants indicated some level of involvement in spiritual retreats. A spiritual retreat represents the type of sacred communal setting that would inherently engage one at both levels of transcendence: (1) intrapersonal in that there is a seeking to know God on a deeper level, and (2) transpersonal in so much as there is a meaning and purpose for participation in the retreat experience in the first place.

In facilitating spiritual retreats, the researcher reportedly engaged participants in some spiritual formation activity involving shared experiences that would ultimately lead to a more meaningful understanding and deeper personal knowledge of God. The researcher's experience has been that most retreat participants were on a quest for meaning; they often talked of knowing about God but not knowing God. Spiritual retreat goers tended to seek a place of sacred solitude to critically reflect on certain religious, spiritual, or life events that have left them dumb-founded (or without a clear sense of purpose). In view of this research, spiritual retreats can be used by adult religious educators as a small group transformative learning opportunity (i.e. spiritual formation).

Additionally, each of the interviewees in this study identified prayer (personal and corporate) as a major coping resource, as did over 75% of all participants surveyed. The very nature of prayer suggests an intuitively transcendent experience—involving some type of reflection focused on problem-solving or expressions of gratitude.

▓ *Demographic Influence*

With the exception of age, there were no statistically significant correlations between demographic variables and religious participation among the African-American women surveyed in this study. Age, education, and income were three demographic factors that created interest in this study. One point of interest was the finding that age had a negative relationship to the experience of stressful life events. The older participants reported fewer stressful life events. A first reaction might be that elderly women are more stable. However, considering the various stages of personal development, elderly women have probably already experienced most stressful life events. My assumptions regarding the relationship between older adults and the experience of stressful life events are that: (1) The house is paid for, (2) children are grown and living on their own, (3) the marriage is stable, and (4) finances are fixed.

Although Houle's (1961) research was not a parallel study, findings from his study do suggest that the use of a heterogeneous sample would yield higher correlations on demographic variables. Houle conducted 22 case studies on a widely diverse group of people who were actively and continuous involved in various forms of adult learning. According to Houle, they varied widely in "sex, race, national origin, social status, religion, marital condition, and level of formal education" (p. 13). A recommendation for future research on this topic is to conduct the survey and interviews on a more diverse population.

In addition to providing demographic data, participants were asked to identify stressful life events that occurred over the last year. For most elderly adults, common life events are likely to have occurred over the span of their life-time, with the likelihood that the older they get, the fewer changes they will encounter. Younger adults would still be in transition when it comes to school, work, and family. Thus, it is my ultimate conclusion that, with the exception of Hurricane Katrina, most elderly women had experienced the type of life events indicated in this study prior to the last 12 months; whereas younger women are still in transition.

The second and third points are inter-related. Although the majority (70%) of the women surveyed had studied at the college level—with 47% holding earned degrees—45% of these same women earned less than $20,000 annually. The disparity between level of education and level of earned income is staggering. Three contributing factors immediately come to mind: location, ethnicity, and gender (i.e., African-American women living in southeast Mississippi). Additionally, all participants involved in this study were also affiliated with Baptist churches, although a few of them actually listed their membership in non-denominational ministries. An empirically-based discussion of these factors requires additional research on the topic. However, it is common knowledge that Mississippi has been ranked as the poorest state in the nation (U.S. Bureau of Economic Analysis, 2006). Economic facts on the status of women, African-Americans, and other minority groups were not researched as a part of this study; however, the researcher assumed that there was disparity in socio-economic status.

▓ *Hurricane Katrina*

Participants in this study reported two major concerns during Hurricane Katrina: family and health (38% combined). Marriage problems, children relocating, living arrangements, and extra persons in the household were dominant family issues identified in this study. Health concerns included personal health issues and health issues of immediate family members. Two participants reported having over 20 people in the same household during Hurricane Katrina. These findings could provide directions for helping agencies as they develop strategies for providing assistance in disaster relief efforts. For instance, more information on family and health issues could be included in disaster preparation plans initiated by church and community organizations.

Adult religious educators could make use of information regarding levels of participation to strengthen program weaknesses. Since participation in religious programming was found to have a positive relationship to coping, programs designed specifically for the purpose of creating transformative learning experiences could be implemented as a preventive measure (e.g., a pastor could direct the congregation in the direction of increased participation in those areas that have low attendance).

Finally, the implementation of church and community programs geared toward building stronger families would serve in the best interest of all parties involved. Healthy women contribute to healthy families; healthy families contribute to healthy churches and communities. If families are healthier spiritually, socially, and physically, they will be better prepared overall during times of cataclysmic disaster. (The low economic status reported by women in this study may serve as an indicator that many of the issues identified were pre-existing conditions; the problems were already prevalent.)

▓ Conclusion

Results from this study are consistent with findings from other studies that support the transformative nature of religious activities on spiritual growth, health, and overall wellness. As can be noted from the interview excerpts, a few of the women reported profound spiritual experiences that transformed their lives in various ways. One participant spoke of loving and accepting others without judgment; another participant focused on reconciling a broken family relationship as the result of suffering such great loss from Hurricane Katrina; still some others dedicated themselves to untiring acts of service.

It is not a debatable issue that Hurricane Katrina was a disorienting dilemma, but so were the rich spiritual experiences that accompanied a few of the conversions that were shared by participants in this study. Meaning-making, reflection, discernment, intuition, and transcendence were found to be prevalent in the stories of interviewees in this study. These key elements exercised within a sacred communal learning context can be instrumental in bringing about transformative adult religious education experiences that are permanent in nature, thus signifying a perspective transformation.

In conclusion, the study found a positive relationship between participation in adult religious education and coping with stress. However a negative relationship was found between age and the experience of stressful life events. Other demographic factors were not significantly related to coping or stressful life events. Results from this study can be used to inform educational programming in both church and community settings. Several recommendations are listed.

▓ Recommendations

1. Repeat this study with African-American women from other denominational and regional backgrounds, as well as those who are non-affiliated.
2. Duplicate this study with men and women of various ethnicity, denominational persuasion, geographical locations, education levels, and socio-economic status.
3. Expand this study to collect addition qualitative data on the role of relationships in the coping process.
4. Expand the concept of this study to explore more closely a cause-and-effect relationship between religious participation and the use of coping strategies.
5. Conduct a longitudinal study to track participants from this current study to assist with developing #4 above.
6. Helping agencies implement more holistic therapeutic and other health related strategies for coping that involve the Bible, prayer, meditation, and retreats.
7. Homogeneity of sample may have contributed to low correlations; use of a random If you answered YES to question three above, which stressful event triggered this change? Will the change be permanent?

REFERENCES

Achterberg, J. (1998). Uncommon bond: On the spiritual nature of relationships. *ReVision, 21*(2), 4-10.

Amstutz, D. D. (1999). Adult learning: Moving toward more inclusive theories and practices. *New Directions for Adult and Continuing Education, 82,* 19-32.

Baldacchino, D., & Draper, P. (2001). Spiritual coping strategies: A review of nursing research literature. *Journal of Advanced Nursing, 34,* 833-841.

Baumgartner, L. M. (2002). Living and learning with HIV/Aids: Transformational tales continued. *Adult Education Quarterly, 53,* 44-59.

Belenky, M. F., Clinchy, B. M., Goldberger, N. R., & Tarule, J. M. (1986). *Women's ways of knowing: The development of self, voice, and mind.* New York: Basic Books.

Belenky, M. F., & Staton, A. V. (2000). Inequality development, and connected knowing. In J. Mezirow and associates, *Learning as transformation,* (71-102). San Francisco: Jossey-Bass.

Billingsley, A., & Caldwell, C. H. (1991). The church, the family, and the school in the African-American community. *Journal of Negro Education, 60,* 427-440.

Bishop, Detra (2006). Adult Religious Education as Transformative Learning: The Use of Religious Coping Strategies as a Response to Stress. Ann Arbor, MI: ProQuest, UMI Dissertation Services Abstracts.

Boudreaux, E., Catz, S., Ryan, L., Amaral-Melendez, M., & Brantley, P. J. (1995). The ways of religious coping scale: Reliability, validity, and scale development. *Assessment, 2,* 233-244.

Boyd, R. D., & Myers, J. G. (1988). Transformative Education. *International Journal of Lifelong Education, 7,* 261-284.

Boyd-Franklin, N., & Lockwood, T. W. (1999). Spirituality and religion: Implications for psychotherapy with African-American clients and families. In F. Walsh (Ed.), *Spiritual resources in family therapy* (pp. 90-103). New York: Guilford Press.

Brant, C. R., & Pargament, K. I. (1995). *Religious coping with racist and other negative life events among African-Americans.* Paper presented at the meeting of the American Psychological Association, New York, NY.

Brown, D. R., & Gary, L. E. (1988). Unemployment and psychological distress among Black American women. *Sociological Focus, 21,* 209-222.

Carey, J. W., Wenzel, P. H., Reilly, C., Sheridan, J., & Steinberg, J. M. (1997). CDC EZ-Text: Software for management and analysis of semistructured qualitative data sets. *Cultural Anthropology Methods, 10*(1), 14-20.

Chatters, L. M., Levin, J. S., & Taylor, R. J. (1992). Antecedents and dimensions of religious involvement among older Black adults. *Journal of Gerontology: Social Sciences, 47,* S269-S278.

Coe, G. A. (1919). *A social theory of religious education.* New York: Charles Scribner's Sons.

Coe, G. A. (1929). *What is Christian education?* New York: Charles Scribner's Sons.

Cohen, S., Kessler, R. C., & Gordon, L. U. (1995). *Measuring stress: A guide for health and social scientists.* New York: Oxford.

Collins, P. M. (1990). Religion and the curriculum: John Dewey and the Dutch catechism. *Religious Education, 85,* 119-135.

Courtenay, B. C., Merriam, S. B., & Reeves, P. M. (1996). The centrality of meaning-making in transformative learning: How HIV-Positive adults make sense of their lives. *Proceedings of the 37th Annual Adult Education Research Conference,* (pp. 73-78). Tampa: University of South Florida.

Coyle, J. (2002). Spirituality and health: Towards a framework for exploring the relationships between spirituality and health. *Journal of Advanced Nursing, 37*(6), 589-597.

Creswell, J. W. (2005. *Educational research: Planning, conducting, and evaluating quantitative and qualitative research* (2nd ed.). Upper Saddle River, NJ: Pearson Merrill Prentice Hall

Culliford, L. (2002). Spiritual and clinical care. *British Medical Journal, 325,* 1434-1435.

Dewey, J. (1933). *How we think: A restatement of the relation of reflective thinking to the educative process.* Boston: D. C. Heath and Company.

Doctor, R. M., & Doctor, J. N. (1994). Stress. In V. S. Ramachandran (Ed.), *Encyclopedia of Human Behavior* (Vol. 4, pp. 311-323). San Diego, CA: Academic Press.

DuBois, W. E. B. (with Gates, H. L., Jr.). (1989). *The souls of Black folk.* New York: Bantam Books. (Original work published 1903).

Dworkin, M. S. (Ed.). (1959). *Dewey on education: Selections with an introduction and notes* (No. 3). New York: Bureau of Publications.

Elias, D. (1997). It's time to change our minds: An introduction to transformative learning. *Revision, 20*(1), 2-6.

Elias, D. G. (1993). *Educating leaders for social transformation.* Unpublished doctoral dissertation, Teachers College, Columbia University, New York.

Elias, J. L. (1993). *The foundations and practice of adult religious education* (Rev. ed.). Malabar, Florida: Krieger.

Elkins, D. N. (1999). Spirituality. *Psychology Today, 32*(5), 44-48.

Ellison, C. G. (1990). Family ties, friendships, and subjective well-being among Black Americans. *Journal of Marriage and the Family, 52,* 298-310.

Ellison, C. G. (1991). Religious involvement and subjective well-being. *Journal of Health and Social Behavior, 32,* 80-99.

Ellison, C. G. (1993). Religious involvement and self-perception among Black Americans. *Social Forces, 71,* 1027-1055.

Ellison, C. G., & Gay, D. A. (1990). Region, religious commitment, and life satisfaction among Black Americans. *The Sociological Quarterly, 31,* 123-147.

Ellison, C. G., & Taylor, R. J. (1996). Turning to prayer: Social and situational antecedents of religious coping among African-Americans. *Review of Religious Research, 38(2),* 111-129.

Ellison, C. G., Boardman, J. D., Williams, D. R., & Jackson, J. S. (2001). Religious involvement, stress, and mental health: Findings form the 1995 Detroit area study. *Social Forces, 80,* 215-249.

Ettling, D., & Hayes, N. (1997). Learning to learn: Women creating learning communities. *ReVision, 20*(1), 28-30.

Flannelly, L. T., Flannelly, K. J., & Weaver, A. J. (2002). Religious and spiritual variables in three major oncology nursing journals: 1990-1999. *Oncology Nursing Forum, 29,* 679-685.

Fontana, D. (2003). *Psychology, religion, and spirituality.* Malden, MA: The British Psychological Society/Blackwell.

Foster, R. J. (1998). *Celebration of discipline: The path to spiritual growth.* New York: HarperCollins.

Fowler, J. W. (1981). *Stages of faith: The psychology of human development and the quest for meaning.* New York: HarperCollins.

Frazier, E. F. (1964). In *The Negro church in America: The Black church since Frazier. The Negro church: A nation within a nation* (pp. 35-51). New York: Schocken Books.

Freire, P. (1970). *Pedagogy of the oppressed.* New York: Harper.

Freire, P. (1973). *Education for critical consciousness.* New York: Seabury.

Fry, P. S. (2000). Religious involvement, spirituality and personal meaning for life: Existential predictors of psychological wellbeing in community-residing and institutional care elders. *Aging & Mental Health, 4,* 375-387.

Gehrels, C. (1984). *The school principal as adult learner.* Unpublished doctoral dissertation, The University of Toronto, Toronto.

George, L. K., Ellison, C. G., & Larson, D. B. (2002). Explaining the relationships between religious involvement and health. *Psychological Inquiry, 13,* 190-200.

Glesne, C., & Peshkin, A. (1992). *Becoming qualitative researchers: An introduction.* New York: Longman.

Graham, S., Furr, S., Flowers, C., & Burke, M. T. (2001). Religion and spirituality in coping with stress. *Counseling and Values, 46,* 2-13.

Groome, T. H. (1980). *Christian religious education: Sharing our story and vision.* New York: HarperSanFrancisco.

Hebert, R. S., Jenckes, M. W., Ford, D. E., O'Connor, D. R., & Cooper, L. A. (2001). Patient perspectives on spirituality and the patient-physician relationship. *Journal of General Internal Medicine, 16,* 685-692. *Oncology Nursing Forum, 30,* 641-647.

Henderson, P. D., Gore, S. V., Davis, B. L., & Condon, E. H. (2003). African-American women coping with breast cancer: A qualitative analysis. *Oncology Nursing Forum, 30,* 641-647.

Hodge, D. R. (2001). Spiritual assessment: A review of major qualitative methods and a new framework for assessing spirituality. *Social Work, 46,* 203-214.

Holmes, T. H., & Rahe, R. H. (1967). The Social Readjustment Rating Scale. *Journal of Psychosomatic Research, 11,* 213-218.

Houle, C. O. (1961). *The inquiring mind.* Madison: The University of Wisconsin Press.

Imel, S. (1998). *Transformative learning in adulthood.* (Digest No. 2 00). Columbus, OH: Clearinghouse on Adult Career and Vocational Education. (ERIC Document Reproduction Service No. ED423426). Retrieved January 27, 2006, from http://www.cete.org/acve/docs/mr00021.pdf

Imel, S. (1999). *How emancipatory is adult learning?* Columbus, OH: Clearinghouse on Adult Career and Vocational Education. (Myths and Realities No. 6). Retrieved January 27, 2006, from http://www.cete.org/acve/docs/mr00021.pdf

Isaac, E. P. (2005). The future of adult education in the urban African American church. *Education and Urban Society, 37,* 276-291.

Isaac, E. P., Guy, T., & Valentine, T. (2001). Understanding African-American learners' motivations to learn in church-based adult education. *Adult Education Quarterly, 52,* 23-38.

Kasl, E., & Dean, E. (2000). Creating new habits of mind in small groups. In J. Mezirow and Associates (Eds.), *Learning as transformation: Critical perspectives on a theory in progress*, (pp. 229-252). San Francisco: Jossey-Bass.

Knowles, M. (1980). *The modern practice of adult education*. Chicago: Follet/Association Press.

Koenig, H. G. (2001). Spiritual assessment in medical practice. *American Family Physician, 63*, 30-33.

Krause, N., Ellison, C. G., & Marcum, J. P. (2002). The effects of church-based emotional support on health: Do they vary by gender? *Sociology of Religion, 63*, 21-47.

Kraus, N., & Van Tran, T. (1989). Stress and religious involvement among older Blacks. *Journal of Gerontology: Social Sciences, 44*, S4-S13.

Lazarus, R. S., & Folkman, S. (1984). Stress, appraisal and coping. Springer, New York.

Leach, M. (1957). *Christianity and mental health*. Dubuque, IO: WM. C. Brown Company.

Leuba, J. H. (1969). *A psychological study of religion: Its origin, function, and future*. New York: AMS Press.

Levin, J., Chatters, L. M., Ellison, C. G., & Taylor, R. J. (1996). Religious involvement, health outcomes, and public health practice. *Current Issues Public Health, 2*, 220-225.

Levin, J., Chatters, L. M., & Taylor, R. J. (2005). Religion, health and medicine in African-American: Implications for physicians. *Journal of the National Medical Association, 97*, 237 – 249.

Levin, J. S., Taylor, R. J., & Chatters, L. M. (1994). Race and gender differences in religiosity among adults: Findings from four national surveys. *Journal of Gerontology: Social Sciences, 49*, S137-S145.

Levin, J. S., Taylor, R. J., & Chatters, L. M. (1995). A multidimensional measure of religious involvement for African-Americans. *The Sociological Quarterly, 36*, 157-173.

Life Application Study Bible (New Living Translation). (1996). Wheaton, IL: Tyndale House.

Lucas, L. L. (1994). *The role of courage in transformative learning*. Unpublished doctoral dissertation, University of Wisconsin, Madison.

Marting, S., & Hammer, A. (1988). Coping resources inventory. Menlo Park CA: Mind Garden. Retrieved November 5, 2005, from http://www.mindgarden.com

Maton, K. I. (2001). Spirituality, religion, and community psychology: Historical perspective, positive potential, and challenges. *Journal of Community Psychology, 29*, 605-613.

Mattis, J. S. (2002). Religion and spirituality in the meaning-making and coping experiences of African-American women: A qualitative analysis. *Psychology of Women Quarterly, 26*, 309-321.

Mattis, J. S., Taylor, R. J., & Chatters, L. M. (2001). Are they truly not religious? A multi-method analysis of the attitudes of religiously noninvolved African-American women. *Perspectives*, 90-103.

McCann, R. V. (1962). *The churches and mental health*. New York: Basic Books.

Merriam, S. B., & Caffarella, R. S. (1999). *Learning in adulthood: A comprehensive guide (2nd ed.)*. San Francisco: Jossey-Bass.

Mezirow, J. (1978). Perspective transformation. *Adult Education, 28*, 100-110.

Mezirow, J. (1990). How critical reflection triggers transformative learning. In J. Mezirow and Associates (Eds.), *Fostering critical reflection in adulthood: A Guide to transformative and emancipatory learning* (pp. 1-20). San Francisco: Jossey-Bass.

Mezirow, J. (1991). *Transformative dimensions of adult learning*. San Francisco: Jossey-Bass.

Mezirow, J. (2000). Learning to think like an adult: Core concepts of transformation theory. In J. Mezirow and Associates (Eds.), *Learning as transformation: Critical perspectives on a theory in progress*, (pp. 13-34). San Francisco: Jossey-Bass.

Mish, F. C. et al. (Eds.). (1999). Merriam-Webster's collegiate dictionary (10th ed.). Massachusetts: Merriam-Webster.

Morgan, J. H. (1987). *Displaced homemaker programs: The transition from homemaker to independent person.* Unpublished doctoral dissertation, Teachers College, Columbia University, New York.

Mulholland, M. R., Jr. (1985). *Shaped by the word: The power of scripture in spiritual formation.* Nashville, TN: The Upper Room.

Musgrave, C. F., Allen, C. E., & Allen, G. J. (2002). Spirituality and health for women of color. *American Journal of Public Health, 92,* 557-560.

Narayanasamy, A. (2002). Spiritual coping mechanisms in chronically ill patients. *British Journal of Nursing, 11,* 1461-1470.

Nye, W. (1993). Amazing grace: Religion and identity among elderly Black individuals. *International Journal of Aging and Human Development, 36,* 103-114.

O'Brien, M. E. (1982). Religious faith and adjustment to long-term hemodialysis. *Journal of Religion and Health, 21,* 68-80.

Pargament, K. I. (1997). *The psychology of religion and coping.* New York: Guilford Press.

Price, D. (Ed.). (1999). Philosophy and the adult educator. *Adult Learning, 11,* 3-5.

Pullen, L., & Tuck, I. (1996). Mental health nurses' spiritual perspectives. *Journal of Holistic Nursing, 14,* 85-97.

Schaller, J. E. (1996). Mentoring of women: Transformation in adult religious education. *Religious Education, 91,* 160-171.

Sealey, J. (1985). *Religious education: Philosophical perspectives.* Boston, MA: George Allen & Unwin.

Siegel, K., & Schrimshaw, E. W. (2002). The perceived benefits of religious and spiritual coping among older adults living with HIV/Aids. *Journal for the Scientific Study of Religion, 41,* 91-102.

Stein, J., Hauck, L. C., & Su, P. Y. (Eds.). (1975). The random house college dictionary (Rev. ed.). New York: Random House.

Szumigalski, S. (2004). Religious problem-solving and locus of control: Coping and controlling. UMI ProQuest Digital Dissertations. Ann Arbor, MI: ProQuest Information and Learning Company. (Publication AAT 3119088)

Taylor, E. W. (1997). Building upon the theoretical debate: A critical review of the empirical studies of Mezirow's transformative learning theory. *Adult Education Quarterly, 48,* 34-59.

Taylor, E. W. (2000). Analyzing research on transformative learning theory. In Mezirow and Associates, *Learning as transformation: Critical perspectives on a theory in progress* (pp. 285-328). San Francisco: Jossey-Bass.

Taylor, M. W. (1990). Harriet Tubman. Danbury, Connecticut: Chelsea House Publishers.

Thompson, J. (2000, March). *Emancipatory learning.* NIACE Briefing Sheet 11. Retrieved January 27, 2006, from http://www.niace.org.uk/information/Briefing_sheets/Emancipatory_Learning.pdf

Tisdale, E. J. (2001). Spirituality in adult and higher education (Digest No. EDO-CE-01-232). Columbus, OH: Clearinghouse on Adult, Career, and Vocational Education. (ERIC Document Reproduction Service No. ED459370). Retrieved January 27, 2006, from http://www.ericdigest.org/2002-3/adult.htm

Tisdale, E. J. (2000). Spirituality and emancipatory adult education in women adult educators for social change. *Adult Education Quarterly, 50*(4), 308-335.

Townsend, M., Kladder, V., Ayele, H., & Mulligan, T. (2002). Systematic review of clinical trials examining the effects of religion on health. *Southern Medical Journal, 95,* 1429-1434.

Tough, A. (1979). *The adult learning projects: A fresh approach to theory and practice in adult learning.* Toronto, OISE.

U.S. Bureau of Economic Analysis. (2006, February). Statistical abstract of the United States, 2006, (Table 662). Retrieved September 21, 2006, from http://www.census.gov/statab/ranks/rank29.html

Vaillant, G. (1977). *Adaptation to life.* Boston: Little, Brown and Company.

Vogel, L. J. (2000, Spring). Reckoning with the spiritual lives of adult educators. *New Directions for Adult and Continuing Education, 85,* 17-27.

Walsh, F. (1999). Religion and spirituality: Wellsprings for healing and resilience. In F. Walsh (Ed.), *Spiritual resources in family therapy* (pp. 3-27). New York: Guilford Press.

Wethington, E. (2003). Life events. In Fernandez-Ballesteros (Ed.), Encyclopedia of psychological assessment (Vol. 2, pp. 561-564). Thousand Oaks, CA: SAGE.

Wiessner, C. A., & Mezirow, J. (2000). Theory building and the search for common ground. In Mezirow and Associates, *Learning as transformation: Critical perspectives on a theory in progress* (pp. 329-358). San Francisco: Jossey-Bass.

Wiley, A. R., Warren, H. B., & Montanelli, D. S. (2002). Shelter in a time of storm: Parenting in poor rural African-American communities. *Family Relations, 51,* 265-273.

Zamble, E., & Gekoski, W. L. (1994). Coping. In V. S. Ramachandran (Ed.), *Encyclopedia of Human Behavior, 2,* 1-10. San Diego, CA: Academic Press.

Printed in the United States
By Bookmasters